Born Naughty
A true biography of the author

Kim Martin

Published by

MELROSE BOOKS

An Imprint of Melrose Press Limited
St Thomas Place, Ely
Cambridgeshire
CB7 4GG, UK
www.melrosebooks.com

FIRST EDITION

Cover designed by Tanya Fukes

ISBN 978-1-906050-72-6

Printed and bound in Great Britain by:
Biddles, 24 Rollesby Road, Hardwick Industrial Estate,
King's Lynn. Norfolk PE30 4LS

This book is a work of non-fiction based on the recollections of Kim Martin. Some of the names of people, places, dates and the detail of events have been changed to protect the privacy of others. The author has warranted to the publishers that except in such minor respects not affecting the substantial accuracy of the work, the contents of this book are true.

Contents

Chapter 1
My Beginning

20 May 1961: the time was 16:30. My mother had just left the restaurant, thinking that she had enough time to go to the hairdressers, even though she had been experiencing labour pains. Suddenly the pain became unbearable and she had to be rushed to hospital very quickly, the pain was me. I could not wait to get into this world, and before my mum could get onto the labour bed, there I was, weighing just 5lbs and scaring everybody. The doctor and nurses could tell that something was wrong. My mum was now panicking as the look on their faces was enough to tell her that it wasn't like this when my sister was born. However at this time they didn't realise the seriousness of my condition.

"It's just a cyst," they said. "It will go away." They sent us home and my parents were left watching me and worrying.

Three weeks later I was growing more and more of a concern to both doctors and my parents, and was taken from my family and admitted into Great Ormond Street Hospital, where I remained critical for several weeks. The doctors had diagnosed me with Spina Bifida. Spina Bifida is caused by problems in the development of an embryo in the womb. It is known as a "neural tube defect" as it results from the failure of the embryo's neural tube to develop properly. The neural tube forms in the first few weeks of pregnancy and eventually goes on to form the baby's brain, spinal chord and their coverings. Spina Bifida is when the neural tube does not develop properly and this results in an incorrectly developed spine. All this information was just too much for my parents to take on board, and they just had to put all their faith in the doctors. By now I was wired up to lots of machines just to keep me alive. I wasn't feeding and it seemed that I had lost the will to live.

"We need to operate," the doctors informed my parents. "This is going to be very risky." They also said that it would probably do damage, but were not sure where. My parents had no choice; my life was in their hands. They did operate, with no obvious damage appearing initially. I fought the will to live and started to feed, yet after 3 months of being in this world I still only weighed 5lbs. My strength did eventually start to grow and I was eventually sent home. This was just the start of my difficult journey into this world, particularly the hospital stay. Life was never going to be the same for my parents, constant worry, protection for me, and also my sister to consider who was three years my senior.

A few months down the line I started to crawl, and my parents' worst fears started to materialise. I was not crawling properly. I pushed myself along on one side, dragging my leg behind me. These were the signs that the doctors had warned about, nerve damage had occurred. Thankfully it only appeared to be my one leg and no other symptoms had been noticed. The endless journeys to the Hospital started in earnest now and this was to shape most of my life, particularly my childhood. The road from my little seaside town to London was hard financially and physically for us all, especially my dad who was trying to work and keep the family together. These trips were every three weeks. I have flash backs of cameras clicking, being poked and prodded, and a mumbling of voices as the doctors talked over me.

The next thing I remember was being in Tadworth Hospital and having my leg broken several times a week. This was done to try to make the leg grow, as it had started to grow shorter than the other one. They had to do it, they said. I was so scared, lonely, confused, in pain, and worst of all, separated from my dear family. "Why are people hurting me?" I did not understand. When the trolley came for me, they took me down the corridor, the long, cold, scary corridor. In addition, I had a mask on my face, the horrible mask that smelt of rubber, and then I would know nothing. When I woke up my leg was hurting and I cried with the pain and fear within me. The nurses were horrible to me, they told me to shut up and put their hands over my mouth. Moreover, on one occasion they force-fed me, which in later life led me to have eating problems.

Accordingly I became resentful and angry. There is one particular occasion that I remember when my mum and dad came to collect me. I was playing with some toys – cutlery and some drawers – when I saw a woman standing at the door. I remember thinking, *I know her* – it was my mum. On getting home I was very emotionally traumatised, I just cried and cried. My parents didn't know what to do. My mum went to the local GP who told her to be very patient with me. He told her that all I had experienced in my life was pain and suffering, and that I didn't understand why, and all I needed was lots of love. He told her, "Take her out in a field and show her the pretty things in life. The flowers, the birds, but most of all keep showing her love and you will regain her faith." This seemed to be the best advice that my mother could have been given. Eventually I started to see that life did have some good things in it and I began to grow and flourish with love.

My hospital visits continued and I was eventually fitted with a calliper to help me to walk. At the age of five I had already missed out on one year of schooling, as the school did not want to take responsibility for my disability. After much-continued meetings and consultations with the school, they finally agreed to take me. Although I only lived a few roads away from my first school, I was provided with a taxi to take me, as they felt this would help my parents and me. I hated school so much. I felt scared, and all the feelings of being away from my family came flooding back to me, just as it was when I was in hospital in those young tender years. I suppose I felt insecure just as I had done when I was lying in the hospital bed.

The smell of the school, I can smell it now, school milk, everybody running round me screaming and shouting. It scared me so much I used to feel sick, literally sick. I was homesick and at night when I was in bed, I used to have nightmares, night after night. The nightmares would be that our house was bombed and I couldn't find my mum, dad and my sister. All I could see was fire and flames everywhere in the street and I was totally lost, not knowing which way to turn. Looking back I think that it was all the insecurities I felt when I was young and away from my family, and here I was again, still young and not understanding why I had to go to school. I know all children go to school, but I did not want to go. My mum used to explain to me that all children had to go to school, and she even had to say to me, *If you don't go then they will take you away from me*. That did frighten me because I had been away so much already, and I didn't want to go again. I tried to go, although often the school would ring up and say, "Can you come and collect her, she has been very sick." My mum or my elder sister would have to come and collect me and take me home. This continued for many more months, right through my early school years. Consequently all I remember are bad feelings, bad memories, and hating every minute of it. Wishing for the bell to ring so that I could go home, longing for the summer holidays and Christmas, when I could spend a long time at home with my family.

The other things I was experiencing between the ages of five and nine were feelings during the night where I would wake up and the room would disappear in front of me. It would go far away in the distance. The curtains and walls would seem to move as if they were stretching out further and further away from me. I used to be so scared and I used to scream for my mum and dad. They would come in, and I would say to them, "I have got that far away feeling again." I had experienced it so many times.

They always said they understood, they said, "Don't worry, we know how you feel. It will go away soon." They would cuddle and comfort me, and make me feel better in their warm love. They were right, those feelings did eventually go away, but I think psychologically it was probably the feelings I had experienced throughout the years of being away, and I was still trying to come to terms with it all.

I continued to go to school even though I hated it. However I made lots of friends, which was a good turning point for me. At that time I was able to walk, run and do all the things that little girls do. Dressing up, playing, looking forward to Christmas, summer holidays, and all the things children enjoy doing in their spare time. I really enjoyed being with my friends, having fun, talking, and although I wore one calliper, nobody ever treated me any different. I also hobbled to one side a little when I walked, but they got used to that and so did I.

Consequently life did get better, I did progress, and I was able to read and write, and do all the things that the other children were doing. Even school sports I could do, such as the egg and spoon race and jumping in the bag sack race. My parents would come along and cheer me on, and I improved. I did have the odd bad day, however. For instance, I remember one day walking up the school steps and tripping up on the step. I had badly grazed all the skin off my good leg, and thinking, "Ouch that hurt." I remember it well. Summing up, my primary school life had gradually improved and I was making good progress.

So there I was, now walking with a calliper, and having lots and lots of love from my parents and having some really good times. In particular Christmas and birthdays and all the things parents love to do for you during these happy times. However, one of the hardest things that my mum had to endure was the fact that I needed constant exercising on my bad leg. If at any time my mum had given up on me, then I would not have been able to continue to walk. Accordingly she persisted day in and day out, even though I dreaded it as it was really hard work for both of us. There were some nights when I was so tired, when perhaps we had been on a long journey to the hospital in London. We would come home, and we would be exhausted, but my mum never ever failed me, and I always managed to do my exercises. Every night she would help and encourage me to do these exercises with my leg to make it strong, and thus enable me to continue to use it with my calliper and walk. My leg wasn't strong enough to walk without the exercises; it needed constant manipulation and movement. At night my mum would have to put cotton wool between my little toes, to prevent them from curling over each other, and wrap my leg in a back slab of plaster with bandages round it so that I could not bend it during the night. These plaster casts had been especially made for me, and moulded to my leg shape. My leg had to be kept perfectly straight, which had to be done every single night, and my mum never ever failed.

The hospital visits continued and we were going up to London on a regular basis. It was always difficult fitting it around school and my parents' work. My dad had a job that he was working really hard at, and my mum was also working while trying to support my sister and me. In between we were still travelling to the hospital to hear the latest news about me. Pictures would be taken of my back and leg, and these would be discussed constantly, regarding what further procedures needed to be performed. Would they leave me this time or would they have to perform further operations on me? Consequently, we were up and down, backwards and forwards to Great Ormond Street Hospital in London. This happened every three weeks and lots of different things were done to me over the years.

My dad tried to make hospital trips as enjoyable as he possibly could, especially as it was such a long way. He always tried to fit in good things so that I would have enjoyable things to remember rather than just the bad. Therefore as I grew older he would suggest that on some days we would go and see some sights in London. I remember really exciting things, like the day we went to the Planetarium and I remember seeing all the stars in the sky. They took me to Madame Tussaud's and all around the wonderful London streets. I saw such beautiful buildings and it was always so exciting. I always felt so secure with my dad, even though London was so hectic and people can be just crazy sometimes. I could always rely on my dad and my mum to be a real safety net. Those were the good things I remember about my hospital trips, my dad always trying to make them fun. Sometimes on the way home we would break down and would be stuck in the middle of nowhere. There were no mobile phones then, and we would not have anything except the car and the dark lonely streets. My mum and dad would be outside trying to fix the problem, yet at the same time trying to make out everything would be all right. They would always try to reassure my sister and me, that there was no problem and not to worry. He always sorted it, we always managed to get home and I always trusted that he would. I even remember one night a police car came past and asked if we needed a hand, and then helping us to get home. This pattern of life continued for a long time between the ages of six and nine.

I want to go back now and talk about some of my Christmases; those were the best days of my life. Even to this day I think I will never ever forget the things that my parents did for me throughout the years of believing in Father Christmas. They made it so real. My parents did not have very much money, but I never ever knew that. My sister and I never had a clue that my parents were relatively poor. They would save all year so that at Christmas time we could have whatever we wanted. Every year as I got ready for Christmas, all excited, I really believed that Father Christmas existed. I remember looking at all the shiny things, the tinsel, and the lights on the tree. I got so excited about Father Christmas coming down our chimney and eating the mince pies that I had carefully left out for him on the hearth. Until one day my sister shattered my dreams and told me the truth, that there was no Father Christmas. I was devastated, I thought, *How can this be?* and my parents even had an answer for that one too. They said to me, "Of course there is a Father Christmas, I am your father and it is Christmas. He gives you the presents doesn't he?" I suppose in a way it all made sense. Subsequently Christmases were still fun with the things that we would do and all the presents we received.

We used to wake up about four o'clock in the morning, so excited, and look around at the bedroom so full – and I mean full – of toys. There would be parcels everywhere, all surrounding the bed and on top of the cupboards. My sister and I would sneak out of bed and go into my mum and dad's room. They would be lying there waiting, giggling under the covers, knowing that we would be coming in. They would set up a tape recorder so that they could record the whole experience for us to keep and thereby play the tapes when we got older. I still have these tapes to this day. My sister and I would be shrieking with excitement, talking to each other loudly, jumping on the bed and dying to open our presents. My mum and dad would get up and sit with us, as we opened them one by one, and I could never believe how they knew every single thing that I wanted. Tiny Tears to a pogo stick, a beautiful dolls' house, everything they could possibly manage to fit in they did. I thank them so much for that as these were really good times in my life that helped make up for the difficult ones that I had before.

Chapter 2
The Years in Hospital

When I got to about nine years old, suddenly everything started to change and not for the better. We were going to the usual hospital visits, only this time the doctors were talking more intensely and more seriously, much more seriously than they ever talked before. I didn't understand why. My mum and dad looked very concerned; they didn't quite know what the doctors were saying. They basically had told them that they needed to operate on my spine. They said it was necessary. They had been looking at x-rays over the years and realised that things weren't as good as they should be. My spine was not forming correctly, and certainly not growing like a normal person's spine, in fact it had started to curve badly. They showed my parents the x-rays and said that if they did not operate soon, the chances were that I would die because my ribs were actually pushing into my vital organs. Although I was not suffering at the time and did not feel any pain, the doctors seemed to be sure that these things were happening to me. Therefore they told my mum and dad that it was very necessary for them to operate, and to do it fairly soon. My mum and dad at the time had faith in doctors, as you do; they wanted everything to be right for me and they went along with it. Within a few months I was called in to a particular hospital many miles from my hometown. This was to change my life forever.

It is now September, the year is 1970, and I am fast approaching possibly the worst four years of my life. The doctors had told my parents that I had to have a major operation on my spine or die, so there we were, faced with this huge decision. We were told at the time that I needed one operation only. This one operation would fuse my spine together. This meant taking a piece of bone from my hip and grafting it into my spinal column and fusing it together so that it wouldn't bend or curve any worse than it had done already. The day before my operation my mum and dad suggested that they take me out of the hospital and go for a fun day out at the nearby Farnborough Air Show.

That was a really lovely treat for me; I was walking around the air show, loving the sights and enjoying the excitement and roar of the planes as they took off. It was also hard trying to understand that tomorrow was a big, big day for me, yet at the same time trying to put it at the back of my mind. I was trying to tell myself that it would be alright, it would be OK, it wouldn't be like the last time when I was little. *I am older now, I can cope, and I can get through this now*. However, the day before, when we had been in the hospital and I had seen my bed, I could not help but start to feel the same feelings I had felt before, insecure, frightened, and even terrified. That smell all came back to me, the smell that I had noticed so many times before when I was young and I didn't understand. Now however I did comprehend, I understood that I was going to hospital to have one operation, that they were going to make me better and I would be able to go home for ever.

My mum had arranged to stay up at the hospital with me for a while, until I had gotten over the major part of the operation, but obviously for personal reasons she could not stay with me indefinitely. No one knew how long I was going to be there, so she was offered accommodation. My mum and my sister accepted the offer and therefore they did end up staying with me to begin with. This did give me some security, even though deep down I was so terrified and I did not know what to do with myself. Subsequently we returned from the Farnborough Air Show and in fact this proved to be the last day that I ever walked in my life.

The day of the operation arrived; this was one day that I will never ever forget. This day changed my life forever and was to leave me in the condition that I now find myself. The doctors came round before the operation as they always did. They stood at the bottom of the bed and they mumbled things to each other, talking about me, not to me, over my head, not even really talking to my parents. They finally said, "We will see you later," and off they went. The next thing I know was that I was put in the bath, scrubbed from head to foot and dressed in a white grown. They put me back to bed and gave me an injection, the injection that made me feel horrible, not so much with the injection pain, but with its effects. It was supposed to make me relax, but in actual fact it did the opposite and made me feel so scared. My mouth was dry and I thought I was going to choke. I just wanted it all to go away so quickly, but it didn't. The next thing I remember was that they came for me with the trolley. "Not this horrible trolley again," I thought, "the one I used to go on so many times before." But it was that trolley, the trolley with the big metal sides that hold you in. They lifted me onto the trolley and they wheeled me down the very long, cold, stony corridor. The corridor was outside, under a covered walkway, and it led along to all the different wards. I remember the floor that glistened; it had shiny slabs that went all the way up to a long big slope that took me on to the operating theatre. We entered the doors and my heart was racing, racing so fast that I could hardly breathe. My mum and dad left me at those doors. As I said good-bye, tears were rolling down my face, I was so scared. "Please don't leave me," I begged, but they had to, they had no choice. My fate now was lying in the hands of the doctors, only they could cure me.

I don't remember very much after that, in fact I didn't remember very much for quite a time. When I came out of the operating theatre I was put into intensive care, where I stayed a few days. Everything in there was a blur, I didn't know anybody, and I didn't know anything. Again I was scared and in so much pain, I can feel the pain now as I write these words. I felt as though my back was going to rip open. They used to turn me from one side to the other, and I would scream in agony, but the screaming went nowhere, nobody listened and nobody could hear me. It was silent, just silent screams for help, for which no one could do anything. The scary thing was, I didn't even know where I was. Everything was so confusing; all the drugs they had given me were going around my head, making everything seem a nightmare. I remember my mum, although I did not realise it was my mum at the time. She did not look like my mum, to me she looked like Hansel and Gretel's mum, with a huge nose, and I could not believe that was actually my real mum. "Get away from me!" I screamed. "You frighten me," I said as she came forward to cuddle me. I did not recognise her, the drugs were confusing me. I was also hallucinating about the room, seeing huge insects on the ceiling. In actual fact I learnt later, it was just a crack in the ceiling. I thought that I was somewhere else; I thought that I was in the middle of a room with a television blaring in front of me. I kept telling them to put me back, put me back up against the wall. I don't want to be in the middle of the room. My mum would try to reassure me that in actual fact I was up against the wall. I do remember one thing, my mum was touching my bed and pointing to the wall, saying, "Look, there is the wall, it's here, you are in the right place, please don't be scared." To me none of it made sense, I could not understand why I felt like I did. It was only days later when I realised that I had been given many drugs that caused me to hallucinate.

Eventually I left the intensive care unit and was admitted onto the ward. Sadly I was admitted onto a geriatric ward and not a children's ward. Why I don't know, whether they did not have enough beds on the children's unit or what other reason there may have been. My very first few hours in there were not good memories. The sister of the ward was a horrible, nasty nurse; she had a small frame and pointed features, and marched around very swiftly in her dark blue uniform and white hat. She took one look at me and immediately seemed to take a dislike to me. I remember her saying, "You have got to eat, and you can't stay on that drip for the rest of your life." I remember her trying to force scrambled egg down my throat as I had not eaten for a few days while I had been so ill. Again I was terrified, I was in pain, and I did not know anything except that I did not want to be here. My mum and dad had a lot of problems, especially with this particular sister on the ward, they complained to her, and they complained about her. Eventually she was reprimanded and we were given a very brief apology by the hospital. I remember being on that ward for quite a while and I was glad that my parents were there with me as much as they could be. The doctors kept visiting me, and the main reasons they kept coming was that when I woke up from my experience in intensive care, I actually could not feel anything in my legs. The doctors would put pins and needles down my legs and say, "Can you feel that?" and "Can you feel this?"

Each time my answer was the same: "No I can't."

"Oh, it is just bruising," they said. "It will come back, you will be OK."

Terror struck over my whole body as I realised that I couldn't feel my legs. What was happening to me, what had they done? They kept trying to reassure us, my parents and me, by saying over and over every day, "It's just bruising, and it will come back." This went on for so long, however, that I felt in my heart something was terribly wrong, and I think my parents thought the same. At the time my back was black and blue from the operation, so we just had a tiny hope that what they were saying might be true. Subsequently, as each day passed and the bruising got better, the feeling in my legs did gradually start to come back.

Not long after the operation, the doctors came to see my parents. One particular doctor, who had performed the operation on me, stood at the bottom of the bed and said, "By the way I am having to hand you over to another consultant because I am emigrating to Toronto." Shock and horror came over my parents' faces, as they listened to his words in disbelief. How could this man, who had performed such a major operation on me, stand there telling us that he was going to leave? He was going to leave me in the hands of another person – how could he do that to us? How could he expect us to accept that he was abandoning us and leaving the country in less than three weeks' time? His decision was final, and he handed me over to another consultant.

A few weeks after the first operation, they began to feel that perhaps the procedure they had performed was not working. I think they were realising that in actual fact they had caused some damage to my spine. Although some feeling had returned I was not able to move my legs. Therefore I was in a far worse condition than when I had entered the hospital. They made another huge decision that they would operate on me yet again. This time the new specialist wanted to try another idea. He said he wanted to insert a Harrington rod into my spine, which he felt would support it. It was a new thing at the time, they had not done many operations of this kind, and I felt at times that I was just a human guinea pig. Looking back now I feel that I was right. Anyway the decision was made, and after a few days all the preparations started over again. Going back down to the operating theatre, only this time I did not have the strength I had before, I was very ill and unable to accept all the decisions that were being made on my behalf. I had no say in it; I had to take it no matter what. My life was no longer mine; the decisions were not even coming from my parents, as they watched me lying there so poorly. They had no choice but to accept every decision that the doctors made.

The night before my operation, my parents arranged for the priest to come and see me. They wanted to get his blessing, because I had no strength, and in fact I was very close to not existing in this world any more. I think my will had gone and my inclination to live and carry on was not there any more. So the priest came and stood next to my bed, opened the bible and mumbled some words, words I don't remember. It all seemed a blur, like he was giving me my last rites. My mum was looking for something, anything that would help me, help me gain the strength that would enable me to get through the next stage of my life. I needed to get through the next operation, praying that this time it would succeed; praying that this time my life would be able to be normal and I could go home. One of the things that really scared me was remembering the pain. I was only just getting over the pain in my back that had slowly eased, which each day felt less and less. Now I had to endure it all again, only this time it was still fresh in my mind. Before, I had been ignorant of what they were going to put me through. I was fully aware that last time the pain had woken me up, and remembering how my back had felt, how the pain was unbearable and feeling as if my whole body was going to fall apart. However this time I was fully aware of what they were about to put me through, and again I had no choice. I was prepared for theatre, given the usual things, the pre-med, and the anaesthetic; although this time I was not even sure if I was going to wake up.

I was in theatre a very long time during the operation, and I don't remember much after I initially woke up. I remember being back on the ward and not in intensive care. I think things had gone a little bit better than the first time. When I woke up I was lying on the bed looking at the floor. I couldn't understand why I should be facing downwards. The reason was that I had been placed in a special bed called a "Striker bed". It was designed so that you were unable to move any part of your body except your arms and head. The width of the bed was literally the width of your body. It was suspended in a metal frame, which they used to hold the bottom part and which you lay on. You were positioned either facing the floor or facing the ceiling. To turn you over they placed an identical part to the bottom, except without the face hole, onto your back. They then strapped you in and turned you over without you having to move a muscle. It was very frightening and scary to have that piece of bed put on top of you, to be lying there totally in the nurses' hands and being spun over either face down or looking at the ceiling.

This was my life now and I had to accept it. The pain gradually eased up again as it did the first time and I was confined to this striker bed for about six weeks. My life consisted of using mirrors, because when you are facing the floor the only way you can see any other part of the ward is to look into the mirror. I found this very easy after a while and was able to direct the mirror towards my visitors or up the ward just to see what was going on. Life was difficult and boring, looking at the ceiling or looking at the floor, but somehow I found a way to get through it. I found the strength to continue without panicking and without too much fear. I knew this was temporary and eventually they would take me off this horrible machine. Finally I did come off the striker bed and was placed into a plaster cast. This cast went from just under my arms to all the way down my body to my hips. At last I was then put onto a normal bed, which I was to continue in for very many months. Again I was used to being on my tummy but this time I was able to move myself. I was able to lift myself up onto my elbows so that I could do things like read and look around the ward. The nurses found that the best way to look after me was to take the head of the bed off and turn the bed round the other way. I was able to have a table at the bottom of the bed, lift myself up onto my elbows and maybe draw, write and even just eat. I was supposed to spend four hours on my back and four hours on my tummy, with this routine continuing day and night as it had been on the striker bed. I still used my mirrors a lot, especially when I was lying on my back. When they first put the plaster cast on, there was a horrible feeling of it being too tight, and I felt as if I could not breathe. I remember saying to them, "I can't breathe," and they said, "Just relax, you will get used to it and that feeling will disappear." They were right, eventually the feeling did subside.

One of the things that I really enjoyed at the time was drawing. I had learnt to draw Mickey Mouse and Donald Duck and I had got this off to a fine art. Every time I met somebody I used to draw them my Mickey Mouse and Donald Duck, sign it and give it to them.

After several months of being like this my parents obviously could not stay with me. My mum and sister had to go home, and life had to begin alone. I made lots of friends while I was in hospital, some dear people that I can still remember today. I was on a mixed ward at times so there were boys and girls, and it was nice to interact with both sexes. We could all have a laugh and some of the things we got up to were real fun. My friends and I used to try and make life as easy as we could. There were several people in the same condition as me, one particular girl I remember, had just had a Harrington rod fitted and she was put on the striker bed, the dreaded striker bed, next to me. I remember talking to her with words of comfort as she started to look around after her operation. I remember saying to her, "It will be alright, Louise, you will get through it, it's not nice but you will get used to it and then you will be like me." I like to think that my words of comfort helped her. I had another dear friend called Julia, and we were together for several months. She did not have the same condition as me; she had problems with her hips, which were in plaster. So between us we used to talk, laugh and draw, and generally play and have fun. Well as much as you can do lying in a hospital bed.

But the sad thing was I met so many people who came and went, and when they went home my feelings of loneliness and despair would strike in again. How was I going to manage without my friends? How was I going to manage when they went home and left me on my own? I watched them pack their bags, all excited that they were going home, after several weeks staying in the hospital. My heart would sink as they walked out of the door. They reassured me by saying I would be next and I hoped in my heart that they were right. I watched their excited faces trying to be happy for their sake. I wanted to be happy for them. I wanted to go home too, but it wasn't my turn. So I waved them goodbye and they reassured me over and over again that they would be there for me, and that they would come and visit me. Some of them did, some of them came round with their parents and bought me things. In fact I was in there for so long, that some of the children would be admitted again at a later date for something else. They would say to me, "Oh, you have been admitted again too," and I would have to answer them, "No, I have not been home at all yet."

The other thing that was hard, was the fact that my parents could only come up and see me every few weeks. However the parents of my friends that I made on the ward would come every day as they only lived a few minutes away from the hospital. They would try and visit me too, and they would often bring me in supplies, sweets, comics and nice treats. That meant a lot to me. I also had a very kind lady who did voluntary work for the hospital. She would visit children like myself whose families lived a long way away. She was a dear lady, very well spoken, kind and gentle. Even to this day I thank those people, if they ever read this book, for the way their kindness came through to me when I was lying alone in my bed.

Seeing my parents was lovely, I used to get so excited. I had a dog at home called Pippa and I missed him. I missed my dog so much that on some occasions my dad would bring him up in the car, but obviously he was not able to come onto the ward. However my bed had a veranda behind it, so sometimes my dad would take Pippa onto the veranda and I could see him through the window. I longed so much to hold him and cuddle him, but it was winter so I was not allowed out onto the veranda. But it was so nice to see Pippa through the window. They would then have to place him back in the car before they visited me.

My old friends, my dear school friends, I missed them all so much. When I was first in hospital, during those early months, I used to hear from them all the time. In fact I remember receiving a massive envelope full of letters and cards from my school and all my class. I would read each one, wishing I were back there, wishing I could be with my old school friends, but it was impossible. It was also impossible for them to visit me as I was too far away. So I used to look forward to receiving the cards and letters, and reading them one by one, and then placing them at the bottom of the bed. Finally after several months and years the cards depleted and became less and less, until finally they would come round with the mail and there was none for me. No letter of hope, no letter of praise, and I realised then that my friends were slowly beginning to forget me. But why should they remember, I was no longer in their life. After so many months and years how could they still want to keep writing? They said everything they wanted to say before, "Get well soon. We are missing you." They were still young and trying to live their lives back home, making new friends, and learning at school. My life was so different, so yes they forgot me, and I had to accept that too.

I had loads of dolls, which I loved and played with. Silly really but I loved playing hospitals with my dolls, it had become my way of life. My life now was hospital and nothing else, the people on the ward were my life now, along with my family when they were able to visit me. I saw the seasons come and go, I remember the summer months when I was allowed to lie out on the veranda, enjoying a bit of sunshine, listening to the birds and the trees. Looking around at the blue sky, that felt nice. I tried to pretend I was on holiday, but it didn't work too well. The reality was that I was lying there in a plaster cast, flat on my back or face down on my tummy. I hated the hospital food, but had to accept it. But I took every opportunity I had to hide or get rid of it instead of actually eating it. If I was outside and I didn't like something, the veranda came in very handy. For instance the mashed potato, oh I hated the hospital mashed potato, it was always so lumpy. So when one day I was out on the veranda, I suddenly realised I could get rid of the food without anybody noticing. Normally when they came round to collect the dinner, and found I had not eaten it all, they would tell me off.

"You haven't eaten it all," they'd say.

"But I'm not hungry," was my answer.

"You have got to eat it."

So reluctantly I would try and force the food in, but I found it so hard. Therefore on the days I was on the veranda I realised there was a way out of being forced to eat that horrible food. I would put it in the spoon and catapult it over the edge of the veranda. When I look back now I laugh, the nurses used to praise me for eating up all my food, and I knew that really I had given it to the birds.

I remember my twelfth birthday in particular. It was made special by the sister of the ward who was a really nice person. She had jet-black hair and quite a stern face, but she seemed to warm to me, she arranged for me to have a party. The ward was long and had about thirty beds in it and as I said before it was mixed. I woke up in the morning and they had put balloons all around my bed. They had arranged special party food and my family were there, my mum and dad, my sister and all the friends I had made on the ward. They were all there. I woke up to them all singing and wishing me happy birthday. Immediately the singing stopped, the ward sister suddenly wheeled in a trolley packed with lovely food. Fairy cakes and a massive cake with my name on it spelt out in twelve candles. My presents, I had lots and lots of presents and one special one from my mum and dad. It was a signet ring with my initials in it – K G – placed inside a heart. I had always loved jewellery, even when I was very tiny. In fact I remember when I was three years old, and my mum had taken me down to the shops one day. I was extremely excited as she had promised to buy me a ring, a little signet ring. I treasured that ring so much and still do today. This day on my twelfth birthday I opened the box and found this beautiful gold ring. I placed it on my finger and it fitted perfectly and made me so happy. All the other presents were lovely too; it was so nice that special day, and one that I will never forget.

After a while of being in the plaster cast, I started to get problems. I wasn't sure what was happening, but I could feel it hurting. Pains were coming from various parts of my body. I could feel a tremendous pain in my hip, and I could feel pain on my side and in my back. I informed the nurses, some of whom were really nice, but some of them did not really have any care in them at all and just told me to cease complaining, and stop being a baby. I remember saying to them continually, "My hip is hurting, what's wrong with me?" and they would say that nothing was wrong; just ignore it, and it will go away. However the pain just got worse and worse, and although I tried to follow what the nurses had told me, it was becoming harder every day. The pain started to become unbearable, it didn't seem right, so I continued to tell them, and again they continued to ignore me. Eventually, after several weeks of being in terrible agony, I made a huge effort to put it to the back of my mind and carry on regardless. Eventually the pain did seem to ease, and in fact my hip went numb.

Christmas was coming now and they promised me that I could go home for the holidays. They said that they would transport me in an ambulance to my home, and I really was looking forward to the prospect. I had now been there for two years, I think I had seen many people come and go and nothing else was in my mind except going home, even if it was only on a temporary basis. So they packed me up and put me in an ambulance and sent me away. My parents had not seen me for a while, prior to this home trip. When I arrived home they opened the door, and my mum looked at me in shock horror. She immediately realised what a terrible state I was in. She asked me, "What have they done to you?" I was not sure what she was talking about. I looked so thin and pale and there was a terrible smell coming from underneath the plaster. My mum had done some nursing in the past, and quickly realised that they had made a terrible mistake in my care. This mistake being that they had ignored my cry of awful pains in my side and that something was badly wrong with me.

My mum contacted the hospital immediately and told them to take me back in, to take the plaster off and find out what was happening. They took my mum's advice and took me straight back to the hospital. On removal of the plaster the doctors and the nurses looked at me in shock, with horror on their faces, as they realised what had happened to me. I was covered in sores, weeping, infected, nasty sores. The pain had become so bad before they removed the plaster that it had gone totally numb; in fact it didn't hurt anymore. One doctor in particular, the one who was responsible for me, picked me up, held me in his arms and cried. He was sobbing, saying, "What have we done to you, what have we done to you?" The reason he was so shocked was that I had actually got gangrene in my hip. I was rotting away and nobody had noticed. This created rather a panic in the hospital, the panic of what are we going to do with her, she is so ill.

I was certainly given the very best treatment after that. I remember them placing me on sheepskin rugs, and putting me on a high protein diet, in fact everything they could possibly think of to help me get better. It still did not take away from the fact that my whole body was covered now in sores. The worst one was on my right hip. The others they could dress and clean and try to cover over, but the one in my hip was a major problem to them. So I was now lying in bed on the sheepskin rugs and being treated like a queen. In those days suing wasn't an option like it is now.

"How are you?" they'd say. "How are you feeling today?"

"OK," I answered weakly. I was disillusioned, with the fact that now I had another problem to face; how was I ever going to get better? How was I going to get better from the first operation on my spine, let alone the gangrene in my hip? I had to continue and take a lot more suffering. Initially it meant that I was taken to the treatment rooms several times a day to have the sores dressed. This created so much pain and agony that they had to place a towel between my lips so that I could bite on it. The gaping hole in my hip was so big now where it had rotted away, that you could see the actual bone. All the flesh around it had disappeared as it weeped and hurt.

They tried so many ways to make it better. They first tried dressing it, which went on for months and months, three times a day down to the treatment room. I felt I was on an execution run. Every time they would collect my bed, and take me down to the treatment room. They would place the trolley to the side of my bed and carefully unpack all the tools, swabs and saline solution. They would then pack the hole in my hip tightly with gauze soaked in special antiseptic solution. Pulling out the old dressing was excruciatingly painful. I learnt a lot throughout those months. I learnt a lot about how to dress a wound, what they put on me, and how they would try and make it better. I tried so hard to be brave. They would come for me, and take me down over and over again. I would go down brave and come back in tears, lying there feeling my hip throbbing. The pain was unbearable, but that was just the start of my journey.

This went on for many more months and all the time the doctors would do their ward round looking at me, talking about me, never to me, always mumbling over me. All the time they would be searching for a method to make my hip better. It was still as bad as it was from day one, there was no sign of it healing, no sign of improvement. The next decision was to try to take me down to the operating theatre on a regular basis to try and stitch it. So off I went again, down the dreaded corridor, the cold stony corridor up to the operating theatre, I can still smell it now, into the anaesthetic room, being put to sleep, over and over again.

Every week the same procedure, they tried to sew it, clean it, and do everything possible. Back to the ward over and over they would say the same words "It's not healing, it's still not healing, we do not know what to do."

This now created a bigger problem than the original problem on my spine. By now I should have been receiving extensive physiotherapy to try and get my legs to work again. But because of all the other problems I had, this was put on hold. The physiotherapists came round, but they were very limited to what they could do to me, because of the gangrene in my hip. I was still very weak and poorly, and I had been laid down now in a bed so long that it was impossible to just stand me up and try to walk. So this made it so much harder for me to get back to where I should have been.

Eventually they made a decision, that I should be transferred to another hospital to have a skin graft operation. Yet again subjected to another operation; a skin graft on my hip. They had tried every other solution, but nothing had worked. So I was transferred to a hospital in Salisbury, where I was put on a children's ward. By now I was thirteen, thirteen years old and put on a children's ward which did not have any curtains around the beds. In the other hospital you could pull the curtains around your bed. Therefore I had to wash and use a bedpan without any privacy. This I hated so much. Also I hated being in a ward with little children running around. I felt I wanted to hide away. I could not escape. I just wanted to pull the curtains round. I also had to have a bed bath, which I had now got used to. It was the only choice there was no other way of washing. But one thing that stands in my mind was having little children standing at the bottom of the bed looking at me. If you can imagine what you looked like at the age of thirteen. I had started to grow, puberty had set in, and now I was embarrassed. I was embarrassed that these other children were in the ward and they could see me. But I did not seem to have a choice. That was it; I had to get on with it.

I was taken down to the operating theatre to have my skin graft. I am not sure what happened on that day, it is all a bit of a blur. I remember going to the operating theatre and going into the anaesthetic room, and remembering that it was slightly different from the other operations I had. By now I had had so many, I thought I had got used to the procedure. But on this particular day, I was gowned up and the doctor came into the room and put an injection into my hand. He then asked me how I felt. I didn't feel like I felt before, I didn't feel that echo sound; the one that pulls at the back of your brain and slowly takes you away. I didn't feel anything, I was still wide-awake, able to talk and look around the room. My heart was racing with fear and he said, "Don't you feel anything?"

I said, "No."

Then he went away and he picked up something else in a syringe and came back and injected that one in my hand, slowly pumping it in. I waited again for that feeling, the one you normally get. You are able to feel it travelling up your arm up to your brain and pulling at your head, taking you away from this world. Yet again nothing. He asked me how I felt. I said, "Nothing." I could not understand. Why was I still awake, what had happened? Had I become used to the anaesthetic? Was nothing going to work on me any more? I didn't know and I was too young to understand. Yet again he mixed up another solution and came over to me and injected it into my hand. That time I disappeared, the echo feeling came, and slowly I drifted away. Unconscious, unaware of anything that was happening to me.

The next thing I remember was being back on the ward, I was not aware of any time, and didn't know if it was day or night. Apparently something had happened to me. After the operation they could not wake me up. I had been in the recovery room for twenty-four hours. My parents had been contacted, as the doctors were concerned about me. When I did start coming round I didn't know what had happened to me, all I knew was that I was very, very ill. Everything was a blur. I had a nurse with me constantly and I was so sick. I was sick every few minutes and messing up the bed. I was unable to tell the nurse how I felt, and I just remember they had to keep moving me to clear it up and change the bed. Every time they moved me I was in so much pain. They had taken some skin off my left leg and had performed a huge graft on my left hip. Removed a whole chunk of flesh and placed it over the gangrene part. I was now wrapped in bandages. I had bandages everywhere. My right leg hurt and so did my left leg. I remember having wedges placed here and there to try and stop my legs from moving. But every time I was sick, it meant being moved and that caused so much pain. The nurses had started to lose their patience with me a little, I feel. One told me off and said, "Stop being sick, this is hard work for us, you are making us change the bed constantly." But I wasn't able to comprehend what was happening to me, I just remember the nurse being cross and I was frightened. I was frightened to wake up, I was frightened of being sick, I was frightened of being shouted at and I was frightened of all the pain I was in.

My recovery was slow after the skin graft, but I did recover daily, and after several weeks I had the one hundred-odd stitches removed. With this I suddenly realised that my body was never going to look quite the same again. Now I was faced with a huge scar – and I mean *huge*. Not only the stitches, not only the scar that goes down my hip, but the scar on my leg where they had taken a huge piece of my flesh and transferred it over to the other side. What was all this about, I thought. I came into hospital to have one operation on my spine and now I was disfigured for life. I now had a huge scar on my right hip, a scar that nobody could make better. An ugly wound that took so long to start to get better. It did get better eventually, but the scar is still there, still a nasty huge memory of the gangrene in the plaster. This gangrene should never have been there. All because they did not listen to me, and called me a baby.

I was transferred back to the original hospital in Hampshire that I was in before. I was now able to start a little bit of hydrotherapy. I used to love that. I used to love to get into the warm pool and feel that warmth around my body. However my exercises were very hard, I completely and utterly lost the use of both my legs. The muscles had gone, my tendons had started to shrink, and it was obvious that the signs were there that I would not walk again. They used to come over to my bed, and would try to get me to move my legs. Gone were the days where I could bend my legs myself, and move them freely. The feeling was there, it had come back slightly, but never the same as it had been before. I used to love trying to move my legs, but my heart would sink when I realised that I couldn't.

Eventually after about four years of being in the hospital they decided one day that I could return home. I think they felt they had done enough for now. Home to what I am not sure, but they made the decision to let me go. However, before I went home, I started the long process of going from being bed-ridden to sitting upright. That was a strange feeling, as the fluid in my inner ear had been used to a lying position for so long, and I had to resume my balance to an upright posture. The room would spin at first, and I felt very sick. This had to be done gradually, but eventually my balance returned. I was able to use a wheelchair in the hospital and I liked this, I liked the freedom of not being stuck immobile in my bed.

One of the things I liked most about my new-found mobility was being able to help other people. I remember going around the ward, going up to people and asking them if they wanted anything. You see, I knew what it was like to be trapped in bed relying on other people for everything. So my heart went out to others that were in that position and I felt I wanted to help them. So many times I had lain in my bed and wanted something, but did not have the heart to ask. I had not wanted to burden anybody. The nurses did their daily routine, but I felt that if I asked them for other things then they would get cross, and not want to do them for me. So I tried my best to keep quiet, even though sometimes I was desperate. Although I did not ask, I did know how it felt to want things. Now I was free in a wheelchair and I could go around to other patients and say, "Can I get you anything? Do you want a drink, let me make it for you," and I would go off and make them a cup of tea and bring it back to them. I used to enjoy that so much that it made me realise what I wanted in life. I thought that I would like to look after people, care for them. Also my desire for medical knowledge was increasing more and more on a daily basis. The one thing in life that I wanted was to be able to look after people. Before I went home, I plucked up courage to ask my doctor a huge and courageous question. They took me into the sister's office and I said, "I have a serious question for you. Could I be a nurse or a doctor, do you think? Would it be possible?"

They looked at me with sadness in their eyes, real sadness. I can see it today. They shook their heads and I realised immediately that they were trying to tell me no. Well I started to cry and I said, "Why not?" and they answered, "Because you couldn't possibly do the duties of a nurse or a doctor in a wheelchair, you wouldn't be able to cope."

I tried answering, "It's all I ever want," but it was a waste of time. They fundamentally thought that I would never be able to fulfil my ambition. I learnt a lot in my time in the hospital, above all I learnt patience. I had learnt a lot of care, a lot of how to love people, and how to be loved, and now I was told that I could not do that work. I wanted to nurse people and make them better. I can remember when I was very, very young, maybe four or five, being out in the car one day with my mum and dad. I put my arms around my mum and I said to her, "One day I am going to make people better. One day when you have got a headache, I am going to go and get you a tablet. I am going to have my own medicine and I am going to make you better." So now here I was, being told face to face by a doctor and sister that my dream in life was not going to be possible. I went home and had to accept it.

Chapter 3
Going Home

The day I got home, I was excited, so excited. All my hopes and dreams had come true (or at least the most immediate ones). I was free now, free from the hospital, free from the smell of the ward, free from the horrible daily routine. I did not have to put up with the hoover and mop going around everywhere cleaning, I was free of the constant hassle and bustle of the hospital environment. Suddenly I was placed into my own bedroom at home. Everything seemed so strange, so small, and so bright; the colours of the bedroom seemed vibrant. I had not really seen colours for many years, not like this, not like my wallpaper and carpet that I had back here at home. Everything seemed so small. I lay in my bed and I drifted off to sleep. I woke up in the middle of the night and it suddenly hit me that I was alone for the first time in years. I was lying in bed and I was all alone. Yes, my parents were in the other room, and my sister was around, but I was in a room sleeping by myself. I could no longer just wake up and glance at the patient next door to me, and ask them a question, or ask them how they were. I suddenly realised that I had become institutionalised. The hospital environment had been so much a part of my life that although I was home I did not know if I liked this empty feeling. I suddenly felt desperately lonely – who would I talk to now, and who would be there for me, who would I play with?

My parents were now responsible for me again. They were disappointed at the way I had been sent home, as the hospital had discharged me bed-ridden with no wheelchair. I have no idea why they did that and I am sure that these days, this would not have happened. But the truth is that back then, that's exactly what they did to me. They sent me home, lifted me onto the bed and left me there. They basically told me that this was it. I could not walk, I could not move around; this was my future.

Prospects for me looked grim. My local GP advised my mum that I should be transferred to a college to learn, as I had missed so much of my education by now. They tried to teach me in hospital at times, I remember learning all the flowers while I was lying in my ward bed. However I didn't learn anything like you would at school. So now the decision was, what do they do with me? I felt a huge burden to society; not to my parents, they were glad to have me home, but to society.

My GP was saying, "Well I think she should be sent to a college."

"Sent to a college," I thought, "I have just come home, I don't want to go away again, please don't make me go away again." But he persuaded my parents that this was the right course for me, and that without this I would have no future and no education.

By now I was becoming stronger, stronger in my mind, stronger in my will, and stronger in the certainty that I did not want to go away. Unfortunately, however, my GP eventually talked me into it, telling me that it was for the best. Reluctantly, my parents agreed. I thoroughly objected, but I went along with it just to prove a point. Before I knew it, I was packed up yet again and sent to a college very near to the hospital that I had just been in and provided with a wheelchair.

When I arrived at the college, I was faced with lots of other disabled people. I found this difficult, as although I was disabled myself, I didn't want to be put in that category for the rest of my life. As I looked around, I thought, "I know I am disabled now, I am more disabled than I have been before, but this is not for me, no way do I want to be treated like this." As I said before, I started to get a very strong will and I said to the college, "I do not want to be here." It was obviously a living-in college as it was too far to travel backwards and forwards from home. I felt as if I had been put in prison, it was even worse than the hospital. At least in the hospital I thought, "I have to be here because I am sick. I have to be here till I am well enough to go home." But being in this college felt like I was trapped, I was not sick now, I just could not walk. I was not meant for this, this was not me. I wanted to be classed as a normal person even though I wasn't. I knew in my mind that I didn't want to be treated as disabled. I lay in bed every morning, ticking off the days on the calendar. They said that they would make me do a trial period for three weeks and I held that in my heart. "Trial period only," I would say to myself, and every day I would wake up and cross another day off. They told me they would review my situation on a weekly basis. Every day they would wake me up and say, "Come along, you have got to go to class." I would force myself out of bed and reluctantly go, thinking all the time that they could not make me do this.

I hated the other children in the school and I think they hated me too. There was one particular day that I remember, when for some unknown reason, one of the pupils who owned a walking stick, wrapped the handle part round my throat. This scared the hell out of me and my throat hurt for days. I hated this environment. I hated the whole thing, everything about it. I did not want this and I was not going to take it. I even had thoughts of running away. I remember one day they let a few of us outside for a while, and I was watching buses go past. I was thinking if I could get on one of those buses I could escape and never come back. But luckily it never came to that.

In the end, I told them outright, I said, "I am not going to stay in this college, I am going home."

They rang my parents and said, "It's no good, we cannot make her stay, and she is adamant that she does not want to be here. If she doesn't want to stay then we can't teach her."

So yet again I was sent home. I was so relieved to be away from that awful place, the prison, as I had come to view it. I was released and both my parents and my GP realised that it wasn't for me. They now had to work out what they were going to do with me. I was back again with no wheelchair to use at home. I used to have to crawl around my bedroom, and to the bathroom. We lived in a small three bedroom house with a flight of about thirteen stairs. I remember these well, as occasionally I would have to crawl up and down them. It was extremely hard and I grazed my legs occasionally in the process. This meant that I picked up sores, which added to my misery.

Eventually my parents were able to get a wheelchair for me to use and keep at home. They actually gave me two, one for upstairs and one for down. Once I got the wheelchairs things became a lot better. My life at that time consisted basically of sitting in my bedroom, being alone, and just having my parents around. My sister was busy, she was out making friends, she had a boyfriend and actually not long after I returned, left home. My parents were going through a very bad patch at that time. I think it was a problem that had arisen, partly because of all the trials that they had gone through with me, all the hospital visits and everything associated with it. They were trying to keep on brave faces for me, while they tackled their problems, but it didn't work. My heart went out to them, thinking some of it was my fault.

I tried to live my life as best I could and my dad installed a television and record player in my room. My life consisted of watching TV, listening to records and drawing. The authorities had arranged for a teacher to come and try to give me one to one tuition. I found this hard, as I did not enjoy it. I did not feel I was learning anything and it was a constant struggle. I tried this for several months.

I did try and find ways to amuse myself while stuck in my room and one way was to sing. I loved the Carpenters and I used to play their records over and over again. Karen Carpenter was amazing, such a beautiful voice. I longed to be able to sing like her, and one day I decided that maybe I should try and teach myself. I would sit down and listen to her records and try to mimic the way she used to sing. Over and over again I would try, until I finally taught myself. It worked, and I felt I could do it. This was a wonderful hobby and I enjoyed every minute of it.

Apart from the singing, I was very lonely living in my room. Sometimes I would go to my parents' bedroom and look out of the window. This had a view out from the front of the house. I could see people walking up and down, and I would see my friends, old school friends that I had not seen for many years. They would wave up at me and say, "Hello, how are you?"

I would say, "I am fine, how are you?"

They would reply with, "We will come and see you tomorrow."

"Really?" I said with hope in my heart.

"Yes, we will come and see you tomorrow, about ten o'clock."

I was so happy and excited that somebody was coming to see me. The next day I had a reason to get out of bed. My friends were coming to see me and I would make an effort. I would get dressed and make myself look pretty. I brushed my hair nicely and I waited, looking at the clock. Ten o'clock came, and no sign of anybody. Half past ten, maybe they were just running late, I told myself. Eleven o'clock, twelve o'clock, and eventually I realised that they had not meant what they said. At the time they had meant it, but why should they bother with me, when they had their own busy lives to lead? They had places to go and people to see. Other old friends of mine even started smoking and had boyfriends, so why would I be important in their lives? Why would they really want to come and see me? I had nothing to say, nothing to offer them, and so I just accepted it. "They were never going to come, were they?" I would tell myself. "What's the point in getting out of bed, what's the point of making all that effort for nothing?"

Eventually my parents said to me that they would transfer my bedroom into the front part of the house, which would give me more space and enable me to look out of the window. They almost made it like I had my own bed-sit. I felt I had a bit more around me than just a bed. I set it up so I had some armchairs that I could turn round and put in front of the bed. Therefore my bed would be in the background and I would have all my belongings around me. I felt a little happier about this and I had the window, the window that looked out onto the main road, and where I would watch the world go by.

Daily I would get ready and look out of the window, and see people walking up and down. On one occasion (I remember it was summer) some boys were walking past. I can't remember how old they were now, maybe fifteen or so, slightly older than me anyway.

They saw me looking out of the window and they shouted out, "Hello, are you alright?"

"Yes," I smiled, waving back.

"Do you fancy going out tonight?" they said.

I was so shocked that somebody had actually asked me out. I shouted back at them, saying, "Sorry, I can't go out."

"Why not?" they asked.

"I can't walk," was my answer.

"What do you mean, you can't walk?" they replied.

"Just that," I said, "I can't."

"Oh, we are so sorry to hear that," and they seemed genuinely concerned. They didn't laugh and they seemed so sincere as they stood there.

They asked if they could do anything to help, to which I replied, "No, I am used to it now, thank you, but thanks for asking, and have a nice day."

They walked away, their faces glancing up at the window, waving back all the time. Blowing me kisses even. I watched as they disappeared into the background. As they got smaller and smaller I saw their waves become more and more distant. They had made my day and they had made me feel so happy. I really felt that they had meant what they said, that they did care and that they would have taken me out. I had never been asked out by a boy before, how I longed to go, but that wasn't meant to be, was it, not in my condition. Anyway the next day, I was in my room and heard a knock at the door. I wasn't looking out of the window on this occasion. My mum answered the door to find these two boys stood there.

"Hello," they said, "we have come to see the girl in the window."

"Oh," she said, "my daughter."

"Yes," they replied. "Is she there?"

My mum came up the stairs and said, "There is somebody here to see you." My heart suddenly started to miss a beat: who could they be? One of my old school friends maybe? Had they remembered me after all this time? Did they feel guilty that they never came to see me and suddenly they thought they should? My mum said that there were two boys stood at the door. "They want to see you, can they come in?"

"Yes of course," I shouted back down the stairs.

My mum let them in and they came up the stairs and into my bedroom and handed me a present. It was a tiny bow containing a ring, which they had bought at the shops after seeing me at the window. They had bought me a present I thought; I can't imagine why anybody would want to do that. But there they were, two young boys caring for me, and that meant such a lot. I placed the ring on my finger and I thanked them from the bottom of my heart. I told them how much they meant to me, as they had taken the time to care, and to call in and see me.

"No problem," they said. "We kept thinking about you when we went and left you yesterday. We wanted to make you feel happy, and we would have liked to take you out."

But I didn't feel that I wanted to go, as I didn't feel ready to face the world yet. I thanked them for their kind offer as I looked down at my shiny ring. It even fitted perfectly and I wonder how they got that so right? They spent a few minutes with me and asked if there was anything else I would like. I replied, "No, but thanks so much for the ring." They explained that they were down here on holiday and were going home tomorrow or they would have called in again. So I said goodbye and I never saw those two boys again. But I will always remember them in my heart as it meant such a lot to me.

After that occasion I think I felt that I needed to move on, I needed to have a purpose in life. I couldn't spend the rest of my time having home tuition, not seeing people, just my parents and the teacher. So I started to get stronger in my mind. I knew now what I wanted and one day I said, "I want to go back to school."

"It's not possible," the authorities told me. "How can you go back to school, they will never accept responsibility for you in a wheel chair."

But I wasn't having this, none of it. "I want to go back to school," I insisted. "If you don't let me go back to school then I refuse all education." I even told the teacher not to come back tomorrow, as unless I went to school I did not want to be taught. So the teacher had to abide by my will, she called at the door the next day, and I turned her away.

Chapter 4
Visit to Lourdes

The loss of the use of my legs was so very hard to accept. One of the things I thought of was, maybe, just maybe if I pray enough and I do the right things, I will be able to walk again. So I used to do funny little things. I would, for instance, cut a piece of paper out, put it between two pages of the bible, hold it up against my chest and say a prayer. I would then go to bed at night, put the covers over my legs and say another prayer. I would hope that in the morning, maybe, just maybe my legs would be normal. I would go to sleep thinking it would all be OK, but I would open my eyes in the morning, frightened. Dare I pull the covers back? Dare I look? What am I going to see? Had it worked? I would pull the covers back only to find that everything was still the same. I was the same as I was yesterday. My legs weren't better.

What am I doing wrong, I thought to myself. I must be doing something wrong. Night after night I would try different things, different prayers, and nothing worked, everything remained the same. I felt a very sinking feeling in my heart; I couldn't lose hope, I just couldn't, there had to something out there that could make me better.

I had long discussions with my parents. "How can I get well again?" I would say. I just wanted them to be like they were before, even though there was a problem with one leg, at least I could walk back then. "We don't know, my love," they would say, feeling so bad for me and wanting my life to be normal again.

One day I was drawn to a film on the television. It was about Saint Bernadette who found the holy spring water. This water was amazing, I remember thinking, and it made people better. This touched my heart so much that I never stopped thinking or talking about it. I sat at the bottom of my parents' bed, full of excitement. "I think I know what will work," I said. "I really want to go to that place, I need that holy water, and I have got to go."

They could see how much it meant to me, and they wanted to help me, but they didn't know how. They did a lot of research and found out that this particular place in the film did exist, and that it was in Lourdes in France. Lots of people travelled there to be healed or in the hope that they would be. Sadly my parents didn't have very much money at the time, certainly not enough to take us to France to fulfil my dream. They were both working and trying to earn enough money to live on and look after me at the same time. Life was difficult for them too. Being in a small seaside town meant that you pretty much knew everyone, and everyone knew you. My dad spoke to a police inspector just in passing one day, about my wish to go to Lourdes. He was so taken back by my desire that he set up a charity for me, asking people to help.

Word soon got around, and before we knew it, people were giving from everywhere. The local TV company got to hear, and came down to film me. So the word spread even further afield, and people continued to give from far and wide. They all wanted to make my wish come true, everyone was backing me, trying to help. My dream seemed no longer to be just a dream, but a reality. I was going to Lourdes. My heart lifted as I felt a whole new wave of excitement come over me, for the first time in many years I felt I had hope, a way of getting better. Everything was going to be OK now. Through all the media coverage and interviews we now had enough money, more than enough. The inspector came round and said we could go whenever we were ready. So all the plans were organised and the big day arrived, the flight was booked, hotel, the lot, everything was ready. All that was needed now was the belief in what I was doing. I had so much faith I thought I was going to burst. I believed that it was going to work, and that I would even leave my wheelchair behind. Leave all that sadness and become normal, like everyone else.

When we arrived in France, sadly I had picked up a flu virus and felt very poorly. My poor mum had to walk the streets one evening to find me a doctor. He gave me some tablets that helped me feel better. We then set off to the Basilica. This is a huge church under the ground, where they all spoke in tongues. I didn't understand a word of it, but I continued to attend anyway. Then the big day came. The day I would be immersed into the holy water, and the day I would be cured.

There were lots of nuns rallying round, and everybody seemed to be excited. There were thousands of people, not at all like I expected. It didn't seem to be like it had appeared on the programme; it all seemed very commercialised. But still there was hope in my heart, even though I did not actually see anybody cured. I was very confused, but I went along with what the nuns said. They took me into this room, where they had these very big stone-cold baths full of freezing water. The nuns took my clothes off, placed a gown into the stone-cold water, took it out dripping wet, and placed it over my body. *Err* that was awful, freezing cold wet gown. But they explained that it would help me get used to the cold before they immersed me into the water. So I went along with it, praying all the time to God. Please God, please God, please let it work. Help me God; I want to get better so much.

I really believed it. I believed that they would put me in the water and it would work. My life now was in their hands, not the hospital's nor my parents', not even mine, but in the hands of God. The nuns immersed me in the water. The feeling was awful as they put me in that stone-cold freezing water. I was trying to be strong and I knew I had to be to do it. I was brave as they immersed me. I can feel it now; I went completely numb with the cold. Was this normal, I thought, maybe this was part of the process that had to happen before I became better. I closed my eyes as they told me to immerse my head under the water. They said a prayer and pulled me out.

I was freezing cold, cold to the bone. I opened my eyes

and looked down at my legs. Nothing different, there was no improvement. My legs looked exactly the same as they had before. "What's happening?" I said to the nuns. "Has it worked, is it going to take a while?"

The nuns looked at me and shook their heads. "Sorry dear," they said. "You obviously did not have enough faith."

Enough faith, I thought, enough faith, what are these nuns talking about? Nobody had more faith than me, nobody, and my heart sunk.

"Come back tomorrow," they said, "and we will try again."

"OK," I said reluctantly.

"Now you must go to the Basilica," they said. "You must pray with all your heart. Listen to the priest, hear every word he is saying and pray to God that you will get the faith to get well."

So I went to the big Basilica Church under the ground where thousands of people sat, and I prayed. I didn't understand the priest who was talking in tongues and different languages. I didn't understand a word of it and neither did my mum. But I did try and listen.

The next day I went back and went through the same procedure as the day before. They immersed me in the water, and they pulled me out with the same result. This went on for several days, and now my heart was beginning to lose all faith. How could they tell me I did not believe, how could they say those things? How could they blame me for this not working? I looked around at all the other disabled people. It hadn't worked for them either. I asked myself, "What faith do you need to have?" I was confused by now, what kind of religion is this?

We went home. I was no better now than I was before, but this time I had to put on a very brave face. I had to tell people about my experience while I was away. I had to tell them how good I felt. But one thing that was really hard for me was that I had to tell these people that it hadn't worked. All the money they had saved for me, all the kind gifts they had given me, had all been a waste. I had to be strong and smile. Again I was on television thanking everybody, thank you for your help and support, but sadly I did not have enough faith for it to work. I found that very humiliating at the time, but I took it, to save hurting anybody's feelings. That was my journey to Lourdes.

There was still some money left over after my trip, and it was suggested that I could buy a cassette tape recorder. In actual fact this was an excellent gift for me at the time, as I was to use it to help me with my singing practice.

Chapter 5
Back to School

I had now returned to my lonely life in my bedroom watching my television and pursuing my love of music. Music had become a big part of my life, as I found it to be an escape from reality. I could lose myself, become totally absorbed in the words, and was able to teach myself more of how each note should be sung. I would do this by singing and recording it, then playing it back. In the beginning I thought how awful it sounded. Over and over again I would keep singing, until I managed to master the art of sounding the same, holding the notes, and mimicking Karen Carpenter. I finally found something I could do that didn't involve needing my legs, or in fact anybody else. It was just me on my own with my music, my records and my cassette player. Perhaps music was what I was meant to live for, I wondered.

Another huge encouragement to me, and my singing at that time, was a young girl called Lena Zavaroni. Her voice was so powerful, she was so young, so sweet, and yet could belt out the songs with the most amazing power. I followed her with great intent, bought her records, and again taught myself how to sing like her, in the same way I had done with the Carpenters. Lena was performing in a town a few miles from me, and it was arranged for me to go and see her. But that wasn't the only surprise, as somehow it was arranged for me to meet her in her in her dressing room. I was so excited; this was the best thing to have happened to me in a long time. I watched her perform the first part of her show, and after that I was taken backstage to meet her dressing room. She was so tiny and shy, compared to how she was portrayed on the television. We talked for a while, and after that meeting we continued to write to each other for a while. She was travelling around the world meeting lots of famous people, and I longed to be able to do that. I kept up my singing in my room, which helped me cope a lot.

After a long time and a lot of persuading the authorities finally gave in to my request to go back to school. They agreed that if my parents accepted full responsibility for me, they would allow me to go back to school for just two afternoons a week. This was a huge step forward for me, although the lessons were only cooking one afternoon and pottery another. Not much help regarding my lack of teaching mainstream subjects like Maths and English etc. But it was a huge step forward to be allowed back into everyday life, and to mix with other teenagers. I was even provided with a taxi to take me there and back. I at last felt normal on returning to school and to be like the other teenagers. Maybe at last I belonged back in the human race, even if I couldn't walk. I was at last out there mingling in and starting to do normal things.

One person, who really helped to change my life, was a girl just slightly older than me. Her name was Jane, she had moved over here from Australia with her family. For some reason she seemed to really care about me and I for her. Nothing was too much trouble for Jane. She would push me around the school in my wheelchair, and we became the best of friends. Even after school Jane would offer to come and take me out in the evening. We would go out to the local youth club and I got to meet more and more friends. Jane was always my favourite though as she had such a kind way about her, and an abundance of patience. Sometimes I would feel for her, as I am not sure all the other pupils accepted her too much. She had light brown hair, shoulder length, and rather a large build. But she had this wonderful personality.

After a few months they closed my Grammar school, and I had to move to a comprehensive. At last the school decided I had managed very well on the two days a week, and therefore decided they would allow me to go back full time. This was just as well, as the new school was ten miles away from home. Again a taxi was provided to take me there and back. The other pupils from my town, including Jane, had to travel by bus. Jane would wait for me to arrive in the morning and look after me throughout the day. We became inseparable in and out of school. Jane was always very clever, she had the most amazing ability to read a book under the desk, but still mange to take in what the teacher was saying. She would always provide the right answers and did very well in her exams. I wished I could have been like that since I had enough trouble just trying to understand what the teachers were saying. But I guess it was because of my huge lack of schooling. I had missed about six years in my life, and therefore I found it extremely difficult to catch up.

Going back to school was a major turning point in my life. It enabled me to make lots of new friends and taught me how to become accepted as a normal person despite my disability. It made me in actual fact a stronger person. I managed after all those years of being in a hospital bed, to find my true personality. I was able to laugh again. But most importantly, I was able to laugh at myself. I was told by my friends that my sense of humour was incredibly funny. I became confident, outgoing, and full of will power to achieve all the things I wanted to.

At this point, like all the other girls in my class, I had started to notice boys. I started to look at them in a different way than I had done before. There was one boy in particular called Carl that I was completely bowled over by. He was the best and most handsome boy in the school. Medium build, dark hair, big brown eyes, and a smile that would make you melt. All the girls liked him and it seemed he always went for the prettiest. I was so envious. He didn't even seem to notice that I existed, let alone go out with me. Not only was Carl at my school, but he attended the same youth club, so my evenings were very starry eyed too.

Jane and I thought up ways in which we could get him to notice me. We found out that he belonged to the choir at his local church. So every Sunday Jane would come to my house and push me the two-mile trip to his church. We would sit there looking so absorbed and interested, but in reality the only interest I had on my mind was Carl. After the service Carl would sometimes invite us back to his house across the road from the church, for a cup of tea. Wow, I thought, back to his house. I treasured every second in his company. Until one day I found out that he had a serious girlfriend, whom he had met whilst she was down here on holiday. So in the end I had to face the facts that I had to move on.

I had started at that point to try to make the best of my appearance. "OK," I thought, "I can't walk, but I should make the best of what I do have." I was very lucky in the fact that I was born with lovely big blue eyes. My hair also was a gift, as people had always commented right from when I was very little at what a lovely colour it was. At this time it was very long with a rich chestnut colour, and natural waves, and therefore it fell nicely onto my back and shoulders. I started to experiment with some make up which gave me a good colour, and made my eyes look an even deeper blue and bigger than before.

Other boys in school were starting to notice me, which I found very flattering, but unfortunately I didn't feel I really fancied any of the ones that asked me out. It seemed the ones that I liked didn't like me and vice versa. Still that's life, I figured.

Back at school I had made other friends, some of whom also enjoyed singing. They used to come around to my house and we would all pretend we were on the stage. I would get dressed up and make the lighting bright by tipping the lamp over on its side. This made the bulb shine brightly on our faces, as we looked in the mirror holding the pretend microphone and signing our hearts out. I would often record these songs on my cassette recorder, so that we could play them back later. To this day some of those friends out there still have the tapes we used. It was such fun, and I was doing one of the things I liked doing best, singing.

My other friends at school had started to play a major part in my life too. One friend was called Debbie and she lived in the same town as the school was in. I often used to stay over at her house, and she would push me to school from there. We built up a very close friendship and are still good friends with each other to this day.

Chapter 6
Saving My Mum

Things at home were taking a turn for the worse. Memories that I wish I didn't have to think about. For personal reasons I don't want to go into too much detail about some of the events at this time, mainly for the sake of my parents' private life. I will only mention but a few. Some of these events could have happened due to the strain and stress of me and my constant ill health. Perhaps they were driven apart as a lot of times my mum had to be away from my dad, and that must have been hard for both of them, being miles apart from each other for months on end. Dad had to manage without his loving wife at home. Likewise mum had to manage without my dad by her side. This must have put a tremendous strain on their relationship, until finally it broke down.

The horrible day came, and I remember it so well. I was in the middle, loving both of them so much. I didn't want to hear the words. "We are splitting up. Which one of us would you choose to live with?" My head was spinning out of control. All my life flashed before me, the good times and the bad times. I felt as if I was being torn apart and I couldn't decide. I did not want to live my life without either of them. But I had to choose, things had happened from which I couldn't escape, and now I had to face the truth.

Looking back now I know things had not been good for a while, but after all the bad things that had happened in my life I just wanted to ignore it and hope it all went away. But it didn't, so the decision was made, dad was leaving us, and mum and I stayed in the house. At this time I was very concerned about my mum, as I did not feel she was coping. She tried to cover over the truth and put on a brave face, but it wasn't working. I felt that my father was not coping either, but he had his reasons for leaving, which I wish not to write about.

I am about to describe one day in my life that is probably going to be with me forever. It was an awful day, a day where I saved my mum's life. I had met a boy at the local youth club the night before. His name was John. He wanted to take me out for the day, so we arranged that he would come in the morning to collect me, and take me out in my chair. When I got home from the youth club, before my mum went to bed, she came into my bedroom and asked what I was doing the next day. I told her about John, and she seemed happy that I had things to do. She didn't normally ask me what I was doing the next day, but I accepted it, and thought maybe she had her own plans. She tenderly kissed me goodnight, and reassured me I would be all right, and off she went to bed.

We had a rule in our house, that if the phone rang and my parents were in I was not allowed to answer it, even though I had an extension in my bedroom. So I always abided by the rule and never picked up if they were home. The next morning I was getting ready for my day out with John, when the phone rang. I ignored it, thinking mum was in bed and she would pick it up. Anyway it rang and rang and rang again. I was getting concerned as mum had the phone just by the side of her bed. I went to the bedroom door and peeped in through the keyhole. The key was in the door, and I could just see a shadow of blue through the curtains, so I knew that they were still closed. With that I started banging on the door and shouting, "Mum, are you there, can you hear me?" There was still no answer. I immediately knew that something was terribly wrong. I grabbed a newspaper sheet and slid it under the bottom of the door. I am not sure how I learnt to do this, maybe I had seen it done on the television or something. Then I poked something through the keyhole to knock the key out, hoping it would fall onto the paper and luckily it did. I then managed to drag the key towards the door and pulled it underneath. It was tight but it came through and at last I could get into the room.

When I opened the door, it did not take long to realise what was wrong. Scattered around the locker was evidence she had taken an overdose of tablets. Then I found a note. My poor mum was lying there unconscious, barely breathing. I took her pulse and found it was beating so slowly. I called the doctor and 999, placed her onto her side and just sat there watching her in disbelief. "What if she dies?" I kept saying to myself. However I did not panic, in fact I remained very calm, almost as if it was not happening to me but to someone else. I then heard the sirens of the ambulance as it raced up our road. "Help is here at last," I thought.

The doctor arrived and the ambulance quickly rushed her off to intensive care twenty miles away. I could not go with her, as the ambulance was not able to take the wheelchair. Also no time was to be wasted in getting her the help she needed. The GP asked me if there was anyone I could go and stay with. I replied,

"No." I was OK and just wanted to be alone to think about what had happened.

I cancelled seeing John that day. Not long after mum had been rushed to hospital, dad came in the front door carrying two bags. "Where is your mum?" he asked.

"She's taken an overdose, Dad," I replied. "She's been rushed to hospital." With that my dad went as white as a sheet, dropped the bags and ran out to his car, speeding off to the hospital as quick as he could get there.

I tried to carry on as if nothing was wrong. I kept hearing the doctor's words going round my head. He said, "Your mum is dangerously ill and we will do our best, but she may not pull through."

I tried so hard to push everything out of my mind, pretending it was just another day. That evening I seemed to go into auto pilot, I even went out with my friends down to the youth club. I didn't tell them what had happened, as somehow, if they had given me sympathy it would have made it more real and harder to shove to the back of my mind. I didn't want sympathy, I just wanted it all to go away and my mum to get better and come home to me.

When I got home dad was already there. He said that mum was stable, but not out of danger. He had already decided that day to come home to us. Mum was finally out of intensive care and dad spent most of his time beside her hospital bed. Mum returned home after a couple of weeks, but of course she was still very fragile.

Chapter 7
Summer Fun

I had been concentrating on my singing and my dad was probably my biggest fan. He believed in me so much. My mum was also taken by surprise at how well I could sing. I remember the very first time they heard me. I was sitting at the bottom of their bed and suddenly burst into singing "Paper Roses" by Marie Osmond. They just couldn't believe it and had no idea I was able to do that. My singing became a regular thing to them, and in fact I probably drove them both nuts, day in and day out singing from my bedroom. My dad had big plans for me. He wanted me to sing to an audience and he set about getting me bookings in different places with different people.

My first appearance was at a place was called Tiffanies, twenty miles from home. It was very posh, with a big stage and a great band. The lights were just how I imagined and it was such a wonderful experience. The nerves got to me at first, but as soon as I started to sing I didn't want to stop. It was an amazing feeling singing to hundreds of people. Everyone clapping and coming up to see me after the show, lots of people wanted to talk to me. I also sang in a wine bar for a friend of ours for a few weeks. However the songs I sang at this place were not ones that I would normally choose; numbers like Connie Francis' "Lipstick on your collar". However I did enjoy it and really got into the swing of things by getting the audience to join in etc.

It used to start in the evening and go on until late at night. This was while my schooling was still in progress and therefore I was finding it difficult to cope with everything all at once. Not long after that, I landed a six week contract for the summer holidays singing in a holiday camp three nights a week. I really enjoyed that. It also meant I could sing my favourite Carpenters' songs, and the audience loved it. Again it was such a thrill to be on that stage singing my heart out. Nothing else mattered at that moment, just me and my music. The bonus was that I was getting paid to do what I loved most. The band was great too and they felt I had more potential.

One evening I was handed a note to give to my dad, I wasn't sure if I should read it as nobody said either way. Anyway after my singing had finished that evening I opened the note and read it. It was talking about London, saying that I had been accepted into a place where I could pursue my singing to a professional level. I was totally confused, why would I want to go to London and sing, I was more than happy with singing here and I didn't want to go away again, not for anything. My life had only just started to stabilise with some normality, my friends, schooling everything was just there for the taking. Why the hell would I want to leave all that right now and work in London? Yet again people seemed to be making the decisions for me. I had had enough of that with my hospital years, so no way was I going to accept this offer. I spoke to my parents about it, and they said they thought that I wanted to be a professional singer. "I do," I said, "but not to go to London and live, and especially when all these arrangements are being done without my agreement." I felt it had all been done behind my back. It was then that I made the decision that if that was what singing meant I no longer wanted to do it. So after my contract ended that summer, I quit singing for everybody, and I did not think I wanted to perform again.

I had made a friend called Jackie who was a sister of another friend I had made at school. Jackie was a lot older than me, but I was always told I had an old head on young shoulders. Maybe it was with what I had been through that I grew up faster, and could get on well with most ages.

Jackie was a pretty lady with blond hair, slim nice figure, and a pretty face. I used to joke and say she lived in my garden, where as in actual fact she lived in a flat that was at the bottom of our property. Our two gardens linked, with just a tiny path between them. She had two young children, a girl and a boy. We became very good friends and most days Jackie would come and collect me and push me around to her flat. She was single at the time, and I think she enjoyed my company as much as I enjoyed hers. We used to have a little signal between us. Her kitchen and bathroom were in full view of my bedroom window. If she was in and wanted me to come around, she would put her kitchen light on. I also would do the same with my bedroom light, and when we caught each other's eye we would turn it off and on several times as a signal. Within minutes she would be at the door collecting me. I would spend hours up in her flat, talking, playing records and sharing our thoughts. I used to envy her a little, as although she didn't seem to have much money or material possessions, she was always very popular, especially with men. I don't know how she did it, but there was always some man there asking her out. Not that I was surprised; as I said before, she was an attractive lady.

On some occasions I would offer to look after her children so she could be free in the evenings to enjoy herself. One evening I remember was jubilee day, and there had been a lot of street parties going on. Jackie and I decided to go out together that evening, and so we both got dressed up and headed off for town. We hadn't been out long when two men started talking to both of us. The one I spoke to was called Daniel, he was about 19 and said he was down here for a while working. We got on well enough, but being so much older than me, I let him take the lead a little as I was still new to being "chatted up". Jackie got on very well with her man too.

The next day Daniel and I offered to baby-sit for Jackie so she could have another evening out with Richard. So off they went and left us alone. I was a bit worried about what to say and how to act, but we started chatting and the evening went smoothly. Daniel came and joined me on the settee, and put his arm around me. I felt a bit unsure, but he kept on reassuring me that it was all right. Next his hands started to wander all over my body. "Bloody hell," I thought, "that felt good, nothing like I have ever experienced before." Then his mouth went over mine, and before I knew it we were kissing intently.

"Do you like that?" he said.

"Yes," I replied, "but I am not sure we should be doing this?" He kept trying to convince me it was normal, and not to fight it. After a while longer I turned to him and said, "We have to stop, as I am too young, and I don't even love you." I pulled away and went over to the fish tank. Jackie had lots of animals. Her fish tank was one of my favourite things in the flat. It was about eleven o'clock when I heard the key go in the door. "Thank God," I thought. "They have come back and saved me making a fool of myself."

I didn't see Daniel alone again after that, and just as well, as we found out he was in a lot of trouble with the police. He had been caught stealing and was awaiting a prison sentence. He did in fact go to prison and he kept writing to me afterwards. However I didn't want to have any more to do with him, as he was getting very nasty and possessive in his letters. That was my first encounter with a man.

Chapter 8
Sexual Awakening

I had a lot of friends, mainly boys a little older than me, and they were regular visitors like me to the holiday camp I sang for. I started seeing a group of eight lads every night. At times we would have such fun, experimenting sexually with each other. I am not sure now how it came about, but I did end up having a lot of foreplay with each one at individual times. I don't think they were all aware that in turn I would, when I had the opportunity, snog and wank them off. In turn I would let them finger me and play with my tits. It seemed it was a secret between each one, only I knew that I had wanked them all off and vice versa. Sometimes it would happen when one of them was still awake and the others were asleep, or if one of them took me home alone.

I started to enjoy these encounters and almost, but not quite, gave in to full sex. Something always held me back from going all the way, it wasn't for lack of them trying or asking, but in the back of my mind I didn't feel I wanted to lose my virginity with someone I didn't love.

It was during this time that I experienced my first orgasm. This was the most fantastic experience I had ever known and it made me want to be very naughty all the time. Then something changed and I started to really care about one of the lads. In fact I became besotted with him. His name was Shaun and he came from Wales. He lived here with his mum, dad and sister. He had fair hair, blue eyes and came over as very funny, always the life and soul of the party. Shaun and I became closer and closer until in the end I realised I had fallen in love with him. I couldn't wait to see him in the evenings and weekends, and life became one big party. I spent more time out with "the gang" as I used to call them, than I did anywhere else.

By now my parents were glad that my life had settled down, and didn't want to put too many restrictions on me. So I pretty much came and went as I wanted, and they never minded me bringing friends home. I was now sixteen. Shaun and I had started to get closer. I loved him kissing me, in fact I never wanted it to stop. We would mess around a lot in company, laughing and joking, kissing and cuddling. Unfortunately I was never able to go to his house, as there were a lot of steps.

One particular night, it was Bonfire night I think, Shaun took me home as usual, only this time I think we both knew what was going to happen. I took him to my bedroom and we didn't really say anything, as we didn't need to, it was obvious. We didn't put the bedroom light on, as my bedroom curtains were still open and let enough light in from the street lamps outside. Shaun started kissing me passionately and I responded eagerly. I wanted him so bad I would have done anything for him. I loved him. I could feel him start to undress me, kissing me gently all over. I could feel his hot breath on my skin, as he lowered his mouth onto my breasts and slid one hand inside my knickers. I could feel myself getting more and more turned on. I had never felt like this before, but I knew I liked it, and I didn't want him to stop. He sucked my nipples and that felt amazing, then he gently removed all my clothing. I was lying there completely naked with his hand touching every part of my body. He removed his clothes, a shirt which I had bought for him a few days before. I remember thinking how he looked so handsome in that shirt. I glanced over to see how excited he was. His cock was hard and erect as he lowered himself on top of me, and in turn I opened my legs in anticipation. "Will this hurt?" I whispered to him.

"I hope not." he whispered back. Then gently he guided his hard penis inside of me, slowly at first, but getting faster and faster. It didn't hurt, I loved every second of it, and I loved him. After a few minutes he let out an almighty gasp, and I felt a hot fluid shoot up inside of me like a bolt of lightning. At the same time I had the most wonderful feeling between my legs and a rush all over my body.

We lay there after for a while just cuddling and talking. I should have been worried that we hadn't used any protection, but I was so smitten I didn't care at that point. Shaun went home afterwards and I slept contented feeling a glow of excitement and love.

The rest of the gang and my parents all knew how I felt about Shaun, although I am not sure if they knew how far I went that night, and many more nights after that. I was however still extremely naughty and I still carried on wanking off the gang while I was going out with Shaun.

Being a seaside town, summers were always filled with holidaymakers, so I got to make friends from all over the country. One of the local girls had started to come to the caravan park on a regular basis too. Her name was Bella, she was a bit younger than me, but we hit it off immediately and she soon joined our gang. She also started to like some of the lads in it. We saw more and more of each other and often Bella would stay over at my house. I didn't really drink, but I knew the gang liked a drink or two, so I would buy some cans in for them, and that way they could come round to my house and have fun if we didn't feel like going out. This became a regular occurrence. It was nothing for my mum and dad to find people crashed out all over my bedroom floor. Bella was really naughty as well and both of us had many sexual adventures, often in the same room but never with each other.

A few months down the line we moved house, from our old place to a new three-bedroom purpose built house. We had been waiting a long time for this event, as we had to apply for a grant, and then wait for it to be built. So the big day came, the sun was shining and things were looking good for our family. The move went well, we had a house-warming party with lots of my parents' and my friends coming, it was fantastic.

School was a bit tricky, I had stayed on to further my education but found it hard. I developed glandular fever, and was very ill for eight weeks, setting me back yet again. I had started to study shorthand, and by the time I was well enough to go back to school, I had missed so much they advised me to drop the course.

One evening at the age of about seventeen, I had been invited to a party. It was a friend of a friend who had been holding the party at their house. It had been a nice sunny day. I remember it well, as I had spent the day on the beach taking in the rays and turning a nice golden colour. My skin isn't dark, but if I do it gradually, I go a lovely reddish brown. This makes my eyes look even bigger and a deeper blue than usual. The colour of my skin toned in nicely with my hair, which was a rich deep auburn and nearly long enough for me to sit on.

I had been lying on the beach with some friends, talking about what we should wear tonight. As it was such a hot summer and the evenings were still warm, I figured I didn't want to wear a lot, especially as my skin was glowing from the sun.

I was asking around what others were wearing, as I knew I didn't know that many people who were attending the party and I didn't want to look out of place. Everyone agreed it was hot and just a small top would be OK. I went home from the beach and ran a nice hot bath, day-dreaming about the nice day I had had, and thinking about what I should put on. I remembered a nice white top I had which was low cut and had some sequins that ran down the middle. I found a pretty white cotton skirt to match, together with white bra and pants. "That will do," I thought as I placed them onto my chest and looked in the mirror. Carefully I did my makeup and brushed my long auburn hair. I placed a white flower hair slide to hold my hair up over one ear. Now I was ready, my lift turned up and took me to the address I was given.

At first when I arrived, I felt a bit nervous as my friend had not yet turned up. It was not long however before more and more people arrived, including some friends. The music was good, really getting people into the party atmosphere and everyone chatted and laughed. Soon I found myself mingling in with people I didn't know and the nerves disappeared as everyone was so friendly to me.

A few hours went by and a lot of my friends had gradually drifted off and one by one gone home. I stayed as I had been in good spirits and made some new friends who showed no sign of leaving. At one particular point I got talking to a man whom I knew vaguely through his working with a friend of my dad's. He was medium build with dark hair, blue eyes and a nice smile. I quickly found out his name was John. "Hi, John, nice to meet you," I said as he sat down beside me, grabbing my hand and squeezing it tightly. We talked for a while and he asked me how old I was. I asked him the same and he replied with, "Thirty one, I hope that isn't too old for you." At this point I remember thinking, "Is he asking me for a date?" My mind was racing over what I would say if he did, when suddenly I could see this woman on the other side of the room looking over at us intently. He didn't falter one bit, and I started to feel uncomfortable as I thought maybe she fancied him and objected to him talking to me. A few moments later the woman came over, and I thought, "Oh dear, this is it, she is going to have a go at me."

How wrong could I have been, she started smiling at me, leaned over gave me a big hug and then introduced herself to me. She said, "Hi, I am Elizabeth," and with that John piped in, "Please meet my girlfriend."

Girlfriend, I thought, blimey and there was me thinking he was going to ask me out. Elizabeth had medium length brown hair, brown eyes, a nice figure and was wearing a very short skirt and low cut top, similar to mine in fact.

She sat down on the other side of me and started chatting away. As I turned to look at her, I felt a hand go onto my leg, I looked down and it was John's hand. I pretended I hadn't noticed and thought he must have made one huge mistake, thinking he had touched Elizabeth instead of me. Elizabeth also looked down at his hand on my leg and just gave me a big smile. I was totally confused by now. "What is going on here?" I thought, scared to look at either of them at this point, in fear of making a fool of myself.

"Do you like that?" she said.

I nearly choked on my drink and replied, "Sorry, what?"

"John touching you," she said with a voice of approval. Oh my god, I thought, this wasn't an accident, he had done it on purpose and it seemed Elizabeth wanted him to.

"I think so," I replied with my heart in my mouth. They both went on to explain that they had been watching me all evening, and that they had both fancied me and wanted to take me home with them for some fun.

I couldn't believe what was happening to me. Was this real? Was it a joke? Do these things really happen? My mind was racing and I was trying to think what I was going to do. The thought had suddenly turned me on a great deal, but I was so scared. What did they want me to do? I had had experience with a man, but not with a woman, and I wasn't sure if I wanted to do this, although somewhere inside me the thought was turning me on. I nodded to them in agreement that I would go with them.

We collected our belongings and quickly left the party, thanking the host on the way out. In the car they sat me next to John in the front seat, and the journey was really quick as they lived only ten minutes away. All the way they were talking to me almost like they were reassuring me it would be OK.

We arrived outside their house and I looked up and noticed a lot of steps. "Don't worry," said John, "I am strong, I can carry you in there, no problem." So I put my faith in his words, and sure enough, with no effort the next thing I found myself sitting on their settee. They offered me a drink, which I accepted, as I thought I may need one to calm my nerves and excitement.

Elizabeth stood up, put some music on and started dancing in front of me. She was a good dancer and seemed to move very sexually in time with the music. A few seconds later, John got up and joined her. I sat there wondering what would happen next. I didn't have to wait long as they started kissing each other right there in front of me. His hands were roaming all over her body, lifting her skirt and grabbing her buttocks. He pulled her into his chest, dancing slower and slower with the music. "Bloody hell," I was thinking. "What is coming next?" Then he started to strip her off, right there in front of me, a few inches before my eyes. She was then just in her underwear and stockings and I could see he was getting aroused. She then started to remove his clothing, revealing his enormous hard cock. His fingers were in her knickers and she was groaning as she stood there. I had never seen another woman's half naked body so close up before and especially between the legs. I hadn't even seen a porn film on the television, and there I was watching it live. They looked over to me, smiling. Then he bent her over, pulled her silky pants to one side and slid his hard cock up inside her.

"Do you like that?" he said.

I gulped and replied, "Yes." This went on for a few moments and they came over, getting closer and closer. Elizabeth leant over and started undoing my top, leaving my white bra exposed to them both.

"Fuck me!" said John. "You've got a lovely pair of tits." They pulled away from their position, him with the biggest hard on I had ever seen and Elizabeth with a very wet pussy, and came and sat next to me on the settee. I knew at that point there was no going back as these two meant business without a doubt. They both started playing with my breasts, with one on each of my nipples and I was really starting to enjoy this attention. They were both sucking and tonguing my tits in an extremely erotic fashion, and it was driving me wild with desire. My nipples were as hard as rocks and I was groaning with desire. John suggested we go upstairs to the bedroom where he said he wanted to fuck me, so he took hold of me and carried me up.

The bedroom was in like an attic shape where the ceiling sloped down on either side. He placed me on the bed and they both started to undress me until I was completely naked. Their hands were all over me and feeling me like I had never been felt before. They seemed so experienced. On the bed there were various vibrators and toys, which they started to use on me. They even both went down on me, sucking and playing with my very juicy cunt.

I found this experience so very horny, but at the same time I was having feelings of guilt. Guilt that people would think I was a lesbian because I had let another woman touch me.

I remember John finally fucking me in front of Elizabeth. She seemed to enjoy that very much as she shoved the vibrator up inside her own cunt while she knelt next to us, watching John's cock sliding in and out of me. Finally she asked him to stick his cock inside her mouth. I watched as she sucked his huge dick. I had never done that to a man before, so I found it fascinating to watch. She licked all the juices from my pussy off his hard cock and told him to come inside her mouth. He loved it. I could tell by the groaning noises he was making while he moved his hips faster and faster towards her. Finally he did it and shot his load into her mouth. She seemed to gag a little and then slowing down removed her mouth from his cock. Remnants of spunk were trickling down her face, as she swallowed it all up. I couldn't believe what I had just witnessed.

We went back downstairs, and I think I was in shock. They took me home, saying all the way how much they enjoyed it and would I like to return, maybe tomorrow or another day. They gave me their telephone number and said, "Please come back as we enjoyed it so much." I thanked them both, telling them I probably would. However I never did, not because I didn't enjoy it, but because I think I was too young to cope mentally with doing something so outrageous.

Chapter 9
Confessions of a Taxi Controller

One of the bosses of the taxi company that took me to school each day offered me a job controlling the taxis. I accepted this offer, as work wasn't easy to find in our little town, especially for me, not being able to walk and access all the buildings. I was grateful to have been offered any job, and figured beggars couldn't be choosers.

So now I had left school, with lots and lots of friends and enjoying a good social life. Things were looking much better. All except for Shaun, whom I split up with after I found out he was trying to get off with another girl who was down here on holiday. Looking back I think I probably loved him more than he loved me. We still remained friends, and the gang still all hung around together doing crazy things.

One of the guys used to have a pet ferret. One night we had a "Lock In" at the local pub, the boys were putting this ferret down their trousers to see who could stand it the longest. Bella and I became even closer, and there was I single and able to do anything I liked. So now the fun began, I didn't see any one man on a serious basis, I just wanted to have fun, and fun is what I had. One of Shaun's friends had always liked me so I had a fling with him; he was a nice bloke, in a way more caring perhaps than Shaun had been. There was nothing serious between us, although I think we both cared a lot about each other. I didn't want to get hurt again so I made it my goal not to care too much or even see someone too often. Bella and I were at one point totally out of control, shagging anyone in sight. We often met blokes down here on holiday, fucked them one day and moved on to another one the next night. We used to joke between ourselves, saying that doing it so often with strangers, we should charge for it like a prostitute, although we never did. We just continued fucking them for free. Sometimes we would meet blokes at the holiday park and go back to their caravan or tent. One night I remember someone shouting "Be quiet!" as I was being fucked in the tent, and obviously making a loud noise from the enjoyment I was receiving. I remember leaving my knickers behind that night, as it was too dark to find them.

So my life had changed dramatically in those few years. I had gone from no life to a free agent, doing whatever I wanted and with whoever I wanted. Most of the company I kept was with men; even at work they were all men. I began to understand how they thought and what made them tick. I did meet a few that I cared about, but things were usually complicated. It wasn't straightforward, for instance they were either screwed up because of a past relationship, or they were still in one and wanted the best of both worlds. Night after night I would meet new people, my life was never boring or dull. I also liked the older men, I am not sure why, but I still feel like that today.

One night I met a man who was in his thirties, he was working at the Lighthouse, and for a few weeks we got on well. One night he arranged to cook me a nice meal up there at the Lighthouse, since it was tricky for him to get out much as he had to keep watch. I turned up in my taxi, and he welcomed me in to a lovely meal. We sat, talked and flirted, and he told me he was married. I didn't feel that this was my problem, as it was him that had to face his wife when he got home. So after dinner he offered to carry me up the stairs of the tower so I could see the massive light.

What fun, I thought, as I sat on a shelf looking out as the huge light went round and round. Suddenly I was aware of his eyes looking down my blouse. I usually wore low cut tops, as I found this was an asset worth showing off. My blouse was white and I wore a white lacy bra underneath. I could feel my nipples getting hard with excitement as he glanced down my front. I swear my nipples were poking through my white blouse. I looked over at his trousers to see a huge bulge. "Come here," I said, beckoning him over to me. He couldn't contain himself any longer, his hands were all over my tits and his tongue was down my throat. We slid down onto the floor and he fucked me for England, right there and then in the lighthouse. I kept wondering if our silhouettes had been shone across the bay for all to see. I saw him for a few weeks after that until he went home.

I did shift work at the taxi office, sometimes starting at 6 am until 4 pm, and other times starting at 4 pm until the early hours of the morning. This was when all the drunks had gone home and the clubs were shut for the night. I preferred the later shift, as I have never been very good at getting up in the mornings. I am naturally more of a night person. I got on well with all of the drivers, but perhaps favoured some a little more than others, and generally they treated me well too. The office had made a deal with me, as my wages weren't brilliant. They offered me free taxis within the town area, whenever I wanted to go out. This was very handy as it saved me relying on friends and family to drive me around.

I am now about 19 and I am leading very much the same lifestyle as the last few years. I still lived with my parents, but I had my own room on the ground floor which had its own private entrance. I had made the room into a self contained bed sit, including having its own little cooker and fridge. So I was very much independent. My mum and dad were still always there for me, but wanted me to have my own space. This arrangement worked well for us all.

You would think that being in a wheelchair would mean that it would be hard to find men to like me. I believed in the back of my mind, it was a stigma that most people would feel. Disability came with some kind of label. However it was never the case for me, and something that I found hard to understand. In fact on the contrary it was nearly always the opposite and some of my friends would also find this hard to understand. Often I would go out with my girl friends to a pub or club, and within a short time, some man would be smiling at me from across the room, gradually homing in on me, and asking for a date. Sometimes my friends would get pissed off with me and would say to me, "It must be because of the wheelchair." We were never sure if this was true and so one evening my friend said to me, "Let me sit in the wheelchair and see if I get chatted up." We swapped places and I sat on the seat at the local club with a drink in my hand, and she sat in my chair, waiting. A man, who was down here working, approached me about an hour later. He came up to me, sat down and asked if I would like a drink, and then asked, "What are you doing tomorrow? Would you like to go out for a meal in the evening?" I felt really embarrassed, as pretending to not be in a wheelchair hadn't worked. I was still getting the same response and my friend said, "Well I don't know, I give up, it's always the same, they always notice you." I didn't understand why, all I knew was that if people smiled at me when I was out, I always smiled back at them, not wishing to appear rude. I always tried to be friendly and perhaps that was the secret.

At work I had started to be chatted up by one particular driver whose name was Fred. He came down here to live after a break up from his marriage. He was a charming man, always knew how to flatter a girl, by saying the right things at the right time. We had started flirting a lot in the office, and he would always be making suggestive comments. If he was working and I was due to be collected, Fred would always offer to pick me up, or he would volunteer to drop me off when I went out. On the way to work he would tell me how nice I looked, gaining my confidence and generally teasing me. He was a lot older than me, but as I have mentioned before I didn't have a problem with this, as I did feel more excited and attracted to the older man. Whilst I was in the office and he was on the road waiting for a job, he would more often than not come into the office and spend time with me. He would tell me how bad things had been for him and his ex-wife and how he had brought his five children up on his own. All these things made me warm to him, and I must admit I started to fancy him.

After a few weeks of flirting and just seeing each other in the work environment, the right moment came for things to progress further. We had both been doing the late shift, and the usual busy time came for the drivers and me, just before midnight. I think it was because people wanted to stay out late, but knew that if they didn't get home before this time the fare doubled. Midnight came and the phones were going crazy. I was giving out jobs like a maniac.

Around 12:45 things started to settle down a little, just a dribble of jobs came through after that. We had to wait around for the local club to close to do the final job, which was to take the club staff home. Fred would keep popping into the office whilst we waited, only this time he was making more than just flirting comments.

He came up close to me, looked me in the eyes with a smile on his face, and started gently rubbing my face. He leant over the desk and kissed me full on the lips, and as his hands started to rub my neck, I could feel myself becoming putty in his hands.

"I've fancied you for months," he said. All of which I wasn't surprised to hear. Then his hands slowly brushed over my erect nipples. "Shit," I thought. "Is he going to take me here and now over the desk?" The office door was unlocked with an open sign on it, and anyone could have walked in on us, even though it was quiet. Often there would still be the odd person wandering around this time of the morning. His mouth was over mine, and his tongue was in my mouth searching every detail. I could feel my heart pounding in my chest. "I've waited so long for this moment," I thought to myself, I think we both had. He lifted me up out of my chair and placed me on the office table, so my legs were spread apart, wrapped around his waist. My skirt was lifted slightly, just up to the top of my legs showing my black panties a little. He was rubbing up and down my leg, getting me more and more excited, when suddenly the phone rang.

I tried to answer it as normally as possible: "Hello," I said. "Taxis, how can I help you?" I swear my voice was shaking as I said the words. It was so difficult to concentrate and it took every bit of strength to keep it together as he continued to kiss my neck. He was giggling at me, as he knew how hard I was finding it.

The voice on the other end of the phone sounded urgent. "Can I have a taxi take me to the hospital?" they said. "I have a sick relative and the hospital has called him in as they're not sure if he'll make it through the night."

"No problem at all," I reassured him. "I'll send one straight over to you." I looked at Fred; he knew the phone call had been urgent, and he was already trying to pull himself together.

"Will you wait for me to take you home after the job?" he asked. "Or would you rather I take you first?"

I had two reasons for waiting, one was I wanted to carry on where we had left off, the other was I was concerned he should get the customer to the hospital as soon as possible. All the other drivers had gone home, as they didn't hang around much after 12.30, especially when it was quiet. So Fred went off to do the job as I waited patiently for his return. I did all the things necessary to close up the office, including diverting the phone to the boss. I turned the open sign to closed, and waited patiently for his radio call telling me he had cleared from the job.

Everything was going through my head, including would I be good enough for him? I thought that if he has fancied me for so long maybe he would be disappointed now. I still didn't have a lot of confidence when it came to fucking someone for the first time. At last his voice came over the radio: "I'm clear at the hospital."

"OK, thanks," I replied.

"Return to base," he answered. "Be waiting at the door."

I turned the lights out and waited for the sound of his car to approach the rank. My mouth had gone dry with excitement and anticipation. My heart was still pounding hard, only this time even faster than before. Why was I so nervous? I had been fucked so many times before. I think it was the build up, it had been going on for so long between us, just flirting and teasing, months of it. Now the moment had arrived, and finally we were going to take it further.

I saw his headlights approach the office and I smiled as they beamed onto my face. I had undone my blouse to the top of my bra, so I was exposing a lot of cleavage as the light hit my face and chest. I wondered if he felt as turned on as I did. He leaped out of the car with the biggest smile on his face. "Come on, darling," he said as he opened the passenger door for me to climb in. I just brushed my hand across his crotch. The evidence was there; his cock was rock hard inside his trousers, as he climbed in and sat next to me. He asked, "Are you ready for this, as I can't wait a second longer?"

"I'm ready too," I replied. He started the engine and drove off.

I wasn't sure where we were going, and didn't really care, as long as it wasn't far. A few moments later we stopped in a very secluded car park. I looked around, it was quiet, there was not a car in sight, and it was a lovely warm summer's night. His hands went all over me, feeling and touching my body. He gently lowered my seat back, so that I was lying down. He started to kiss me again, only this time even more passionately than the time in the office, kissing my neck which I love so much and working his way down to my bra. I remember thinking it was a good job I had worn my new underwear. I had gone shopping the weekend before, and treated myself to a lovely black lacy push up bra with matching panties. The bra made my tits really bulge out over the top. He really loved this, and concentrated a lot on my breasts, touching them, looking at them, and sucking on my nipples. It felt so good lying there in the car as he devoured me; I had waited so long for this moment.

After a while, on treating my breasts as if they were the crown jewels, he slowly went on to lowering his hands onto my wet panties. I responded by lifting my legs up onto the dashboard and opening them, so he could place his fingers between the gusset of my pants and my juicy pussy. It felt so good, I was tingling all over with a warm rush of excitement from head to foot. I started to undo his shirt as I wanted to feel his hairy chest against my breasts. With that he undid his flies on his trousers, releasing his hard cock. Gently but frantically, he climbed on top of me. Suddenly I felt his hard cock entering my wet pussy. The excitement was too much for me to bear, and with that first thrust of his cock I came. Gushing my wet juices all over his cock and moaning in ecstasy. A few moments later it all became too much for him as well, and he couldn't hold back any longer. His back arched and he grunted loudly, "I'm coming," and I felt the hot rush as he exploded his spunk into me.

He then just lay there on top on me with his hot breath on my neck. He cuddled me for a moment before climbing back into his seat. "That was better than I had imagined," he said. "Phew," I thought to myself, I was glad after all that waiting it was as good for him as it was for me. This was just the first of many sexual encounters I experienced with Fred.

Chapter 10
Meeting Patrick

Life had started to settle down a great deal and I was happy with my social life and work. Although it was not the best job in the world, it was at least a regular income for me. Some of the people I had made friends with were down here on holiday. So after they returned home, we would stay in touch and very often I would go away to stay with them. I had one good friend who lived in Gloucester and often I would spend many a week up there meeting her circle of friends, going out to parties and enjoying myself. Life was never boring or dull and if I wasn't here I would go up to Redhill in Surrey and spend some time with another friend.

One day I was at a friend's house locally, when I met a man who was going to change my life forever. My friend's cooker had broken, and she called out a guy called Brian to have a look at it, as he was the owner of the house which she was renting. My friend and I were in the kitchen, chatting, when Brian knocked on the door. She answered it and Brian came in accompanied by another younger man. The other man had dark hair, medium build, green eyes, a rather a cheeky smile and good sense of humour. Brian said, "This is Patrick."

I said, "Hello," and smiled, and both my friend and I decided to go into the other room and leave them to fix the cooker.

Every few minutes they would shout through requests to us, saying "Where is our cup of tea then?" I didn't comment, as it wasn't my house and my friend didn't seem to want to go and make them one, so we both ignored them. After a while they left, saying that they had fixed the cooker. We both commented on why it had taken two of them to fix the cooker. We thought that perhaps they had fancied the idea of a cuppa with a couple of ladies, rather than doing any work.

About a week later, I had gone to a local pub for the evening and I was at the bar talking when suddenly my chair handle was knocked by someone. Looking up to see what had happened, I noticed the face looking down at me was one I recognised.

"Oh, sorry," he said.

"That's OK," I replied. "It happens all the time."

With that he said, "You were up at that house the other day when Brian and I came to look at the cooker."

"That's it," I thought. "That's where I've seen him before."

"Oh yes," I replied. "Sorry about the tea, only it wasn't my place to make you one."

He laughed and said, "We were skiving and thought if you made us a drink we could stay longer as it was raining. We were in the middle of a painting job so we were at a bit of a loose end."

"Ah," I replied, "we wondered if it was something like that."

Patrick and I didn't stop chatting for the rest of the evening. He had been in the Army, but had recently left, and had come down here from his hometown in Wiltshire. He was here about six weeks, performing decorating work for a friend of his brother-in-law. He told me he was staying at his sister's house. I remember thinking to myself what a nice man he was and before I knew it, the time had come for the pub to close. We then moved on to a local club and continued chatting. Patrick offered to take me home after the club closed and I accepted his kind offer willingly. I lived about a mile from the club and he kindly pushed me to my door. It wasn't an easy road as it has a lot of hills, but he didn't seem to mind. We stayed outside for a while, as it was a nice evening. I thanked him and told him how much I had enjoyed his company. He said the same and then asked, "What are you doing tomorrow evening? I don't have any plans at the moment. Would you like to go out again with me?"

I replied, "OK, great," and I gave him my phone number. I

was working the next day, but knew I could be finished early if I wanted, as I was sharing my shift with another lady who liked to do more hours as she needed the extra money. Patrick kissed me goodbye and said he would come and collect me tomorrow at eight.

That night I couldn't sleep as I kept going over all the things we had talked about. It was crazy to think of all the people I had met before, and yet this one seemed different to me. Straightaway I knew there was something special between us.

At work the next day, I had my head in the clouds thinking about Patrick and our next date. "What shall I wear? Will he turn up? Did he really want to see me again?" The strange thing was that I didn't usually mind if I didn't see the same person again. However I hadn't felt like this since Shaun and that was a long time before. I had liked some of them but never in this way.

Eight o'clock clicked over, and I was all ready, looking out onto the gate at the end of my garden. It was dark and my heart was beating faster and faster, when suddenly a figure appeared at the gate, opened it and started walking towards my door. It was Patrick. He was actually here. I opened the door and greeted him with a big smile.

"You look nice," he said.

"Thanks, you too," I said, feeling a little nervous.

I collected my bag and off we went, heading towards the town centre. He joked that he hadn't been used to pushing a wheelchair until last night, and I complimented him by telling him he was a good driver. Patrick was twenty and hadn't yet passed his driving test. However our town was so small that it didn't really matter if he did not drive as nothing was too far away. The only problem was all the hills.

We stopped by a pub called the Anchor as it looked warm and inviting. I was never into drinking alcohol, but just felt happy to be in a pub with lemonade. Patrick liked whisky, and I remember thinking, "Yuk, I don't even like the smell of it let alone drinking it." I didn't feel I needed to drink to be happy, in fact people often thought I had been drinking when I hadn't, as I was usually outgoing and full of fun when out with my friends.

We hadn't been sitting there long when my sister walked in. She was introduced to Patrick and likewise. Then she whispered to me, "Where did you find such a good-looking man?" I shrugged my shoulders in a way to say, "I don't know, but I think I am very lucky," and then laughed. We had a great night and continued to see each other every evening for the next few weeks. Patrick accepted more work, offered by Brian, to decorate a block of newly built flats. I was happy, as it meant he was staying down. He had already said he liked living here, and providing he had work, was happy to stay.

Patrick and I got closer and closer. He had even started to stay over at my place night after night, rather than going back to his sister's. I remember when he would ask me, "Shall I stay at yours tonight?" A feeling of happiness would come over me with the thought that I had him with me all night. We had my room, which as I said before had been turned into a bed-sit with a cooker and fridge. I liked the fact that he started to leave his belongings behind. I had got used to him being with me, used to doing his washing, making his sandwiches for work in the morning, and having him come home to me after work. His sister had also accepted that he wasn't there much, although she never really said anything.

After a few months Patrick said to me, "Shall I just move in with you?" I was delighted and so excited, and that day I spent all day cleaning the room, sorting out drawer and wardrobe space. Even though there wasn't much room, I knew we could manage. My parents didn't mind at all, as they also had become used to Patrick being there all the time by now. They didn't really trouble us too much, as they wanted to give us privacy as much as possible. We all had to share the bathroom, but if we didn't want to spend time with them we didn't have to, as we had our own room and entrance.

Later in the afternoon the telephone rang, it was Patrick. "I don't have to move in," he said, "I've found myself a flat down the road." My heart sank, I was happy for him, but disappointed for me, as he had said on the phone "for him" not "for us". Maybe I had made a mistake, I thought, maybe when he comes in tonight he will say, "I want you to come and live there with me too." Time ticked on, and it was time for him to arrive home, but he was late and I kept waiting to hear him come through the door. Eventually he walked in, but he had been to the pub on the way home. I didn't make a fuss, and was waiting to hear the news on the flat. I had heard him correctly on the phone. He sat there all excited, saying he had found a flat, he was moving in and there was no mention of me. I tried to sound happy for him but my heart was feeling sad. I was confused as I thought we were happy together. I didn't think he would want to live on his own after us spending so much time together. However I was wrong, he did. That night he kept talking about nothing else.

He collected the key and we went round to the flat. It was a one-bedroom place, clean with a small kitchen and bathroom. One thing I noticed was the bed; it was only a small single divan. I said to him, "Will I be able to stay here with you?"

He answered, "The bed is only a single, so it could be tricky."

My heart sank even lower. "Oh, does that mean I can't stay then, what about if I brought a sleeping bag, maybe I could sleep on the floor or a put up bed?"

"Maybe sometimes," he replied. Well there is my answer, I thought to myself. The truth is that now he has his own place, he doesn't want me around.

After looking around the flat, we locked up and decided to go down to the local club, which was still open. I remember sitting there, pen and paper in my hand, trying to help Patrick decide what he needed to buy from the supermarket. He didn't at that point have a clue on cooking, so I tried to make a list of things he may need. Little things that can easily be forgotten like salt, pepper, vinegar, sugar etc.

A few weeks passed by and Patrick had stayed in his flat on his own. On the odd occasion I would stay round there in the sleeping bag on the put-up bed, and every now and then he would stay at mine. Sometimes he would promise to come and stay with me, telling me he would be home at eleven as he was going out for the night with his friends. On those nights I would not be able to sleep, as I was conscious he would be home any time. I would eventually drift off and wake up at about 4 am looking over at the clock. I would start to cry and ask myself, "Why hasn't he let me know he isn't coming back? It doesn't take much to ring someone does it?" Morning would arrive properly and the bed would be empty, and then I knew he had not come home. Later on the phone would ring and it would be Patrick. "Sorry I never came back last night," he would say, "but you know how it is." Sorry was all I ever heard. This happened more times than I can remember.

On one occasion a few weeks later, I was staying with him at his flat. I always had a thing about unzipping the sleeping bag and checking it, as I had a fear of spiders. I didn't fancy getting in it to find a spider running up me as had happened once before, and scared the shit out of me. As I unzipped it, something did fall out, but it wasn't a spider, it was a peanut! What I couldn't understand was how it got there. I asked Patrick if he had slept in my sleeping bag, even though I couldn't imagine why he would need to. He said, "No." So I asked if anyone else had slept in it and he denied all knowledge. That night I had a bad dream that a woman had been sleeping in my bed. The dream was so real. I woke up in a bit of a panic, but kept it to myself, as it wasn't fair to accuse someone over just a nightmare.

We used to regularly use a pub called the Black Swan. Working behind the bar was a woman called Clair and I knew she used to like Patrick. I often caught them giggling and whispering together when he went to order. Again I tried to ignore these things as perhaps I didn't want to face the truth. "He is still with me," I would tell myself even though I was feeling very unhappy. Finally another blow came to me when Patrick announced he was going back to his hometown to work for six weeks or so. I was devastated. He didn't know how long for, or even if he would be going back for good.

The awful day came and Patrick left. I found it so hard not having him around; life seemed so meaningless. At that point I actually knew what the meaning of the word lost meant. I carried on as much as I could, we spoke on the phone, and he would tell me how he was going out with all his old mates. This worried me, as they were not the best influence in the world, and they all loved the booze and the women. I kept putting it to the back of my mind, and thought if he still loved me he wouldn't do anything like that to me. My mum and dad knew how hard it was for me to not see him, so they suggested we take a day out to visit Longleat, and pop over to where Patrick was working and surprise him. So off we went, and I didn't tell Patrick over the phone as I wanted surprise him. I thought he would have been happy to see me, as it had been a few weeks. I got dressed up and off we went.

The day at Longleat was great, and I was so excited about seeing Patrick. We pulled the car up outside the house where he was painting and knocked on the door. Patrick answered, but the look on his face was horrified, not happy at all. "What are you doing here?" he said.

"I've come to see you, I thought you'd be pleased to see me as it's been a while," I replied. My parents left us as and we talked in the living room. I could tell he didn't want me there; it was there in his face. He looked at me with such anger and coldness in his eyes. "I won't stay," I said, and with that wished him goodbye and left.

The journey home was awful and the road seemed to go on and on, horrible bending twisting roads. I don't think my parents really knew what to say, as they could see the situation the same as I could. So they said very little. I sat in the back with tears rolling down my face, every bad thought I had ever had about our relationship was there staring me right between the eyes. Why hadn't I taken the hint before? Stupid me!

The next day I went to work and a friend asked if I would like to go out with her for the evening. Why not, I thought, I have nothing to lose. So I got dressed up as much as I could in the frame of mind I was in, and went out.

Later on in the evening I was approached by a nice looking man of about twenty-one, he had fair hair, blue eyes and was of medium build. He told me he was a fireman in Leicester and had come down here on holiday. He was very complimentary towards me and had a kind nature. I was not my usual bubbly self, but he still seemed interested and asked if I would like a drink. We chatted all evening and eventually ended going back to my place. He started paying me a lot of attention, making me feel wonderful, which was something I hadn't felt for a very long time. He kissed me and I responded, and after a while we went to bed and made love.

Afterwards I felt so awful, and I confessed to him the problems I was having with my relationship with Patrick, that is, if we still had a relationship. I told him I still loved Patrick and that maybe it was wrong of me to have slept with him. I felt I had used him, and now I hated myself for it. He couldn't have been nicer, telling me he understood and saying that he would be here for me if I wanted him. Even though he lived a long way away, he gave me his number and told me to call him anytime. The next day he called to see if I was OK, and he asked if he could come and see me. I said no at first as I didn't want to sleep with him again, but he assured me it would be just as a friend. He came up and we just talked, telling me not to worry and that things would work out for me. I thank him to this day for his friendship.

Two weeks later Patrick rang me and said, "Guess what, I'm coming home." I was so happy. The day he came home, we were lying on my bed talking, he seemed so different, much more loving, and he started to tell me how girls he had met in night clubs weren't like me. I wasn't sure what he meant, but took it all on board. His sister had told him she had seen me out with another man. Patrick asked me about this and I told him I had met a fireman. I felt very guilty and full of regret. Part of me loved Patrick still and part of me was wondering if I should finish with him, as I was not sure I could take any more hurt and rejection. But as I said before, he was very different today, much more loving and caring.

A week later we went to stay with a friend of his near his hometown. Patrick had now passed his driving test so we could travel around. That weekend I had been very ill with period pains, but tried to carry on and not be a spoilsport. But my period that week was the worst I can remember. However we managed to get through the weekend and had a nice time. This was the start of us becoming close again.

Chapter 11
The Marriage

A few weeks more had passed and Patrick and I had been seeing each other for a year. I was at work one day when suddenly I came over all faint and weak and nearly collapsed. My friend at work called Heather, jokingly said, "Hey I feel like that sometimes, but I'm pregnant, maybe you are?"

"I couldn't be," I thought, "I'm on the pill, and have been since I've been seeing Patrick." The signs were not looking good, my boobs hurt like hell, I felt sick every morning, and felt tired constantly. I had all the symptoms. I made a doctor's appointment, thinking perhaps there was something more sinister behind this feeling, and maybe I had cancer or something.

I went to the doctor's on the Thursday, and had the usual blood test and urine sample etc. He said, "I am sure it's nothing," and I believed him. Then Friday morning the phone rang. "Can you come in and see the doctor as soon as possible please?" the receptionist said. "We can fit you in tomorrow." Tomorrow, I thought, what the bloody hell have they found for them to want to see me so soon? That was it; I was convinced they had found something terribly wrong.

Patrick couldn't take me that Saturday as he was in the middle of a job, which had to be finished. Therefore my friend's husband took me down to the surgery. When I got there and saw the doctor sat looking at me, "OH DEAR," I thought, "it's bad news."

He said, "Well I am not sure if this is going to make or break your weekend, but you are pregnant."

Those words came out like a cannon ball. "What?" I replied. "How did that happen?"

"I think you know that by now," he joked.

"No, I mean I thought I was on the pill."

"Well," he said, looking through my notes, "I see here you had a throat infection a few weeks ago, and you had some antibiotics, they can stop the pill working."

"Blimey, I didn't know that!" I responded, nearly falling off my chair. "How do you think I'll manage?"

He replied, "Well, because of your disability I can't say for sure, but I will put you onto a good specialist who can monitor you every inch of the way."

I left the surgery shell shocked, but so happy, as deep down I thought I wouldn't be able to have children. When I arrived home my mum was standing at the top of the stairs and when I told her the news, she nearly fell down them. She cuddled me, and said, "Oh darling, I am so happy for you that you are able to have children." My dad was delighted too. Now I had to ring Patrick at work.

"Are you sitting down, Patrick? We're going to have a baby," I said excitedly down the phone.

I could hear him dropping the earpiece of the phone and screaming with joy, "Really, are we?"

"Yes, yes, yes!" I shouted, and he said he would get home as fast as possible. That news made it one of the best days of my life.

A few days after the news Patrick came home from work and asked me to marry him. I said no at first as I didn't feel it was the right thing to do, because we were having a baby. He said it isn't just that, but he was talking to his boss at work and that he had told Brian that he wanted to marry me anyway, but wasn't sure what to say. I said yes, but from that day to this felt it was for the wrong reasons. I had loved Patrick and I had wanted to give my whole world to him. But I think he destroyed a lot of that in the early days with his lack of commitment and insensitivity.

We had to decide on a date quickly as I was six weeks pregnant already, and didn't want it to look too bad at the wedding.

Therefore all the plans were made hurriedly for our big church wedding. I had to borrow his sister's wedding dress, as I couldn't find one in a shop to fit me. Both our parents worked hard on the reception plans, which were to be held at a local hotel.

The 18th of December was the big day. Dad made my dream come true by hiring a wonderful white Jaguar to take me to the church, and proudly gave me away in front of all our family and friends. Although I was four months pregnant, things seemed to run smoothly. I said my vows and Patrick repeated his. We went to sign the register and when I looked round Patrick was crying. I thought he was regretting it already, but he said it was an emotional moment for him. Everything went to plan (except for my poor granny who fell down the hotel steps and broke her leg). I was now a married woman.

We had to carry on living in our room for the time being until the baby was born and we could be re-housed. My hospital trips for the baby were going well, the doctors said they would like to do an amniocentesis to make sure the baby was all right and didn't have signs of Spina Bifida. So I had to go along with their decision and this was performed shortly after we got married. It involved taking some fluid from inside the womb and testing it. The pain was awful and the test itself was not without risks. They said there was a chance this procedure could cause a miscarriage. After it was over I was told to stay lying down for 24 hours. The next day I was worried in the morning as I had started to notice some spots of blood, but I rested as I was told to. It did settle down and I was back to normal the next day.

The wait for the results was hard and stressful. We had to wait a few weeks as some of the tests were not conclusive until four weeks after the test. I remember it so well, I was so stressed thinking what if something is wrong with the baby, what horrible decisions I might be made to make. They had warned me that if there was a problem they would advise an abortion. What a horrible thought and terrible decision this would be.

I was probably so hard to live with whilst we waited as each day passed, getting closer to hearing the truth. Eventually the phone rang after the four weeks were up and it was the hospital asking us to go in for the results. "It's good news," they said, "the baby is well and normal." We were so relieved and they asked if we wanted to know what sex it was. We both wanted to know and they told us we were having a little girl. I was delighted as I had always thought I would like one of each, but liked the idea of a girl first. I had always looked at little girls' dresses and loved the idea of putting her hair up in pigtails or plaits with ribbons. We were both so relieved that all the waiting was over and everything was normal.

The next few months flew by, the nurse would visit and do all the checks on me and baby, all was good, no problems to detect. I was feeling OK and strong. It's funny, I think pregnancy can give you an inner strength. I remember being at home alone and decided to turn the bedroom around, dragging all the furniture here and there as if I was super woman, thinking I could manage it. When I looked around I thought, "Oh dear, what have I done?" I was stuck in the middle of the room in a mess and I had run out of steam.

Patrick came home to find me crying my eyes out. "What ever are you doing?" he said looking at the chaos. I explained what had happened, thinking he would be cross, but he wasn't. He said I was stupid for even thinking about doing that, even if I wasn't pregnant.

We didn't have any money at the time as Patrick only had a few jobs and was classed as my carer which only gave us enough to live on. We couldn't afford new things, so we had to go to second hand shops or wherever we could find what we needed for the baby. Some people were kind and gave us clothes that their babies had grown out of. We were grateful for anything. We found a pram, an old blue thing, but we scrubbed it up and got it ready for her. I was due to go in on the 23rd of May and have a Caesarian birth. The hospital had said that was what they thought would be best for me.

On Saturday the 21st of May, Patrick and I allowed ourselves a little treat. He had bought a bottle of cider for himself and some sweets for me. We sat cuddled up and watched our favourite programme that evening, and went to bed about 11 pm. In the night I started to get pains, thinking it was trapped wind at first, and I didn't want to keep Patrick awake so I tried turning over. The pain got worse by the early morning and it was clear from other signs that I was in labour, and had been for hours. We rang the hospital, and the ambulance came straight over to take us the twenty-mile trip to the hospital. Patrick was trying to shove bits and pieces into a suitcase, including the last few coppers we had. We were expecting to go in on the Monday and nothing was ready.

The hospital was good with me; they broke my waters and kept wiring me up to machines. The pains came quicker with fewer gaps in between. Each contraction got stronger and faster, but at least this time the pain I was suffering would be for a good reason, and one I would never forget. I didn't want any painkillers, as I thought I wanted to try and do this with a clear head. Instead I asked if they could play me George Benson on a cassette player and as I sang along the pains increased more and more.

Patrick and I kept saying to each other, we are going to meet her today, our little baby, it was such a nice feeling. In fact Patrick got very emotional. Our baby girl was born at 4.25 pm weighing 6 lbs 13 oz. She was so beautiful with a tiny little face, fair hair and pale skin. She was so delicate, yet perfect in every way.

It was all over, mum and baby doing well and after a few days we were allowed home. It was a scary feeling driving home with our baby in the back. Suddenly we were left responsible. I felt like I was borrowing her at first, but eventually we got into the routine. After a couple of weeks we were offered a one bedroom flat fifteen miles away. It was a nice enough flat, but it was stuck out in the middle of nowhere. There were lots of houses, but only two shops and a garage which closed down soon after we moved. The local people were not at all friendly, and I hated every minute there. During the summer of 1983 it was extremely hot and I found it difficult away from the seaside. I would ring up every day to see if they had any properties available back in our hometown. Six months later we were still waiting.

Our finances were so low we could hardly afford the petrol to travel the small distance to visit our families. We didn't have a washing machine either, so on a Monday we would make a trip back to see the family and get the washing done.

Patrick and I had a few problems in those first six months. There was one day I will never forget when Patrick and I had fallen out, although I don't remember now what it was over. I had been over to the only friend I had in this town, and when I returned he was gone. I was shocked to find no sign of our baby, my records were all over the front room floor, and his drawers were empty. I felt despair as I thought he had taken our baby girl as well. I was in such a state, I couldn't even remember my parents' or in fact anyone's phone number to call them. I just sat there, looking at the walls, feeling so desperate and miles from anyone that really cared. How could he do this to me, and I cried and cried, wondering where they both were. A few hours later the phone rang, it was Patrick. "I'm in Maidstone, Kent," he said. He was once based in the army there and wanted to go back.

"Where's the baby?" I yelled. He said he had not taken her and she was with a neighbour. With that my heart was so relieved, as at least I hadn't lost her. Patrick said he was so sorry and drove back to us the next day.

Another month went by and I was doing the usual calling to the council to see if they had a property, and this time they did. A two bedroom flat just up the road from my parents' house, I was so happy. We moved in there as soon as it was ready and Patrick and I were so glad to be back. Our life together did settle down, Patrick was and still is a good dad, and he never minded getting up in the night to look after her.

We decided to take in a student to help us financial-wise, it wasn't much more difficult than feeding the three of us, and our daughter was able to sleep in our room in her cot. We had lots of students come from all over the world. It was a pleasure to share our home with some of them, and teach them English.

Being by the sea, nearly every day Patrick would push our daughter and me along the beach front and into town and back. He was still very fit from his days in the army. Slowly we managed to get the money together to decorate our home and really make it ours. One night Patrick had some very sad news, one of his friends had been killed in an accident. He had been walking home in the dark wearing dark clothes, and a car had not seen him on the edge of the road. Patrick took this badly and I tried hard to comfort him as much as I could, but we were both so shocked.

The hardest thing Patrick and I had between us, was his lack of communication, he didn't always find it easy to say how he felt. Many times it appeared as if he wasn't interested in what I had to say at all. Our interests were so different, he liked football and I hated it. I liked medical things and he hated that. Sometimes I felt we were so unsuited that I believed if it had not been for our daughter we would not have entertained getting married. Therefore at times I think we both had to suffer each other.

The next year we did our best to look after our daughter, as having us both at home meant she had a good start to her life and the attention that little children need. She was such a good child almost as if she was born with a lot of common sense. This was good as having a mum in a wheelchair wasn't easy at times. I had to pick her up differently from other mothers. If I was alone with her and asked her to do something, she would do as she was told and not play me up. I had to show a lot of discipline in my words, as it was all I had to make her understand. If I said no, I had to make her believe no was what I meant. This worked.

We were coping, with the student's money, but occasionally the taxi company would ask if I could cover a shift as well. That meant extra money and with Patrick being around to look after our daughter, this was possible. In some ways it worked better, as it was easier for him to manage looking after her than for me for obvious reasons.

A short time after this I had started to feel rather strange, tired and sick, all the symptoms that I had clearly had before, only this time I didn't think I was ill. I bought a pregnancy test on the Sunday morning and found I was pregnant again. There was the blue line clear as a bell. I was so shocked trying to remember how this could have happened, as we thought we were careful, but it was obvious we hadn't been. Patrick and I were pleased and he said, "Well we have coped with one so we will cope with two." Patrick really did love our daughter so much and the thought of having another child didn't upset him at all. But I was scared, scared that I wouldn't be able to cope, scared that I was now going to be responsible for bringing two people into this world. Scared if something should happen to Patrick, how I would cope alone with two small children. That night I went to bed placing my hand over my tummy, feeling that perhaps I had been irresponsible in some way, that I shouldn't have let it happen.

I went to the doctors and went through the same procedure as before. I was referred to the hospital, and again offered an amniocentesis, only this time I said no. I felt different this time. Before, I had been unaware of the complications, so I had agreed to whatever they suggested. This time I felt more confident since I had done this before. Everything was OK last time, why shouldn't it be this time, I thought to myself. Patrick and I talked it over and both agreed that the only thing you would achieve from having the test was to be persuaded to have an abortion if things were not right and neither of us wanted to do that. We put our faith in things and I kept telling myself, "If something isn't right with this child nature will do its thing, and if it doesn't then all will be fine." That is what I believed.

Each week I grew bigger and bigger, felt more tired and sick 24/7, much worse than the first time. All the hospital visits were good, the scan showed nothing bad so things were looking good for us. My addiction to cream was out of control, poor Patrick. One night he went down the local restaurant to get me a cream cake as I had such a craving.

The nine months passed very quickly, and the day came to meet my second baby. It was 17.05 on Thursday the 17th of June.

"It's a boy," they told me as they wrapped him up and placed him in my arms. I was half asleep, but I remember thinking how wonderful it was to hear those words. I had a little boy and my second wish had come true. We named him Simon. Now I had one of each, the perfect family. Patrick was the happiest man, so proud to be holding his little son. He chose the name this time as I had chosen my daughter's.

All our friends and family gathered around the bed congratulating us. He was such a cute baby, dark hair, and dark skin, in fact he looked just like his dad. We took our son home and settled him in. Our daughter loved her new brother, and being the little mother she was, tried to help, by fetching things if I needed them.

Patrick was always very good with our children and he would always cope better than me at getting up in the night. I didn't sleep well as I had a problem with my nose. I had been prescribed a nasal spray many months before with blocked nasal passages, and to cut a long story short had become dependent on using this spray. I was dependent on the spray day and night or I couldn't breathe at all through my nose and even went deaf. So this was a major problem for me both day and night. Grabbing sleep whenever I could to catch up was essential and therefore Patrick would take over looking after them as much as possible. It took two operations on my nose to eventually sort this problem out. After such a long time of suffering, I was so relieved to be able to sleep at night and breathe properly.

Chapter 12
The Rod

The children were growing and doing well, my son Simon was aged six months and my daughter was two and a half. I had woken up one day to my back feeling very sore. It seemed worse when I moved, a bit sharp even, as though something inside was touching the skin. The soreness got worse and worse that lunchtime. I remember making some soup, as we all liked my homemade carrot, potato and onion soup. I was sitting at the cooker stirring this soup, holding my back and wishing the pain would stop. Patrick walked past and I said, "Can you just have a look at my back for me and see if you can see anything?"

As I lifted my top Patrick let out an almighty gasp and said, "Oh no, what the hell is that!"

Poking out of my skin was the top of the Harrington rod that had been fixed to my spine when I was ten. About half an inch of the rod had pierced my skin, and this was now protruding out. Patrick wasn't one to overreact, in fact usually he would be the opposite and try to brush over things by saying nothing, but he went white and said, "Don't move, I'm going to ring the doctor."

"What is it, what's happened?" I said, and he replied, "Your rod is coming out and I think it's best if you stay still."

I was scared and the children were looking at me as tears rolled down my face. "This is major," I thought, and suddenly all my past hospital life started to spiral in front of me. All those bad memories from when I had the rod inserted all those years ago. I kept remembering how everything had gone wrong, the gangrene, the years of being away, and now I looked at my kids, thinking, what if all that should happen to me again, only this time it would be much worse as I wouldn't see my lovely children.

Patrick explained the situation over the phone to the doctor, and the doctor said he would need to ring a hospital and get advice, as he wasn't too sure what the situation would be. He knew it was serious but had to get superior advice on where to send me as soon as possible. After about half an hour he rang back and advised Patrick, "I have arranged for an ambulance to collect her and she will be admitted into casualty at the hospital twenty miles away. They will decide from there what is best." He also mentioned that he didn't want the ambulance to take me until he had got there as he wanted to supervise.

It was all panic stations. I couldn't move, so Patrick had to pack me a case and deal with everything. The ambulance pulled up and put me on my side on a stretcher. The doctor turned up, looked at me and handed the ambulance driver a note to give to the hospital. Off we went and I was waving bye-bye at my children, feeling so desperately scared that I wasn't going to be back for a very long time. I was so scared that this would all go wrong again for me.

Pulling into the hospital A & E department they put me into a private room, where several doctors came to examine me and I had x-rays taken. Hours and hours I was in there lying on a trolley worrying what they were going to do to me. It got to about eleven o'clock at night when the doctors decided they would admit me to a ward. The consultant advised me they were going to take me to the operating theatre as soon as possible, as they were worried that infection may start and spread down my spine. He explained they would cut the top of the rod off and it should be all right. I breathed a sigh of relief as maybe it wasn't as serious as I had thought.

So in the morning I was prepared for theatre. Usual procedure, experiencing that echo feeling as they put the needle in my hand, and losing control of my mind as the anaesthetic took over my body. The next thing I remember was waking up in the recovery room. My back was sore, but not as bad as it had been before. I rested in bed and Patrick brought the children to see me. I only had five stitches. "What a fuss about nothing," I thought, and the next day I was sent home.

After the stitches dissolved the scar wasn't too bad. I carried on as usual, thinking it was all over, when suddenly the pain came back with the same sharpness just like before. I knew this time however what was happening and knew it was the rod again. The doctors said this time it would have to come out completely as it wasn't going to be as stable as they had previously thought.

I was now sent to a hospital fifty miles away. My parents were so worried about me, as they were not confident the doctors would know about these rods. The doctor who inserted it had now gone private, and was working in Essex. I found this out because my mum had been so worried about it, that she had tracked him down desperately seeking his advice. He was most concerned on hearing the news about the rod coming out on its own. He also asked if it was at all possible for me to go to Essex, as even though he had now gone private, he would perform the rod removal operation at no charge. This offer was very kind of him, but I was still very worried about going all the way to Essex, as I still had a lot of hang-ups about going into hospital at all, let alone travelling two hundred miles away from my home and children. I didn't accept his kind offer, and decided to stay with the original NHS team, as this involved going only fifty miles to another hospital.

I was admitted there within a day. The surgeons advised that they would take the rod out completely, but not entertain the idea of inserting another one. They said it was far too risky with my spine being as fragile it was. I accepted their opinion and was so worried, in case it all went terribly wrong. Just taking the rod out was very dangerous as it was fixed to the spine with hooks and pieces of wire. What they couldn't understand was why or how it had moved so much on its own.

I went to theatre and was in there a long time as they performed the delicate operation. As they put me to sleep so many thoughts went through my mind. One was "Will I be paralysed when I wake up?" I was scared and looking back I think the doctors were too. Patrick and the children came and stayed near the hospital for a week to be with me, which was great.

I woke up feeling dreadful and in a lot of pain. "That's a good thing," I remember thinking. "That means I am not paralysed." The operation had gone well and I was sent back to the ward with drips and drains everywhere. That day was a bit of a blur, and I was as white as a sheet from the trauma. However I did go to sleep in the end.

The next morning the doctors were concerned as I was still losing a lot of blood. They came around my bed, huddled together with their stethoscopes and white coats, murmuring to each other. Again it seemed they were talking about me, rather than talking to me, "Just like before," I thought, "when I was a child and history was repeating itself."

"What's wrong?" I said, lying there flat on my back at their mercy and looking very white as I felt the blood drain out of my face.

They came closer and replied, "It's nothing to worry about." Although they tried to reassure me they still had a look of seriousness on their faces. "You are anaemic and with all the blood loss we need to give you some iron through an intravenous drip, or you could be going out in a box!" I was horrified, as I felt OK apart from the obvious pain.

In the end I made a miraculous recovery and two weeks after the operation I was allowed to sit back in my wheelchair and push myself around as before. After three weeks I was discharged. No one really knew why the rod had come out, or if I would be the same without it. Doctors did mention it could have been through carrying the two babies, but I felt it was worth it. Even if that was the case I would do it all over again to have my two dear children.

Chapter 13

Problems with the Marriage

Just after the ordeal with the rod coming out, we had managed to find a house with three bedrooms. It needed a lot of decorating and work but we thought it would be worth it. We needed more room now the children were getting older. It was slightly harder for me, as we had a flat before and now we were in a house with stairs. I had a stair lift fitted, with a wheelchair at the top and one at the bottom. The children had a bedroom each, and Patrick and I managed in the little dining room downstairs, so we could still take in students. I was working more for the taxi office again, and Patrick had decided to go back to his trade as a decorator. The only down side to this was that our son was handed to a child minder most days and with Patrick not there, it was hard for me to mange to look after him, especially in a house. Our son also found this hard and he often cried when he was dropped off. Looking back I think we both feel guilty about the fact that our daughter, who had just started school by now, had both of us in her earlier days, whereas our son did not.

Life was becoming more hectic, juggling around work, students, and now we had taken in three lodgers. They did shift work for an oil company so were with us at staggered times. Meal times and shopping were crazy and most days I was cooking for eleven people. However that was not the hardest part, it was more the fact that our kitchen was also being refurbished and this was making life so difficult. All the work tops etc. were being taken out, and new ones put in.

Patrick had got into running, he enjoyed it, and he got fitter by the month. He was even running half marathons and occasionally full marathons in different towns over many weekends. This meant a lot of training every evening and sometimes up to three hours a day. The children and I would often go along and support him, in all weathers.

I had started to go out in the evenings, sometimes with a friend. With it being such a small town, it didn't matter if you went out alone as there was always someone to talk to. I found this a form of relaxation, getting away from all the mundane chores at home. I suddenly felt I had a reason to get dressed up, and something to look forward to. It helped me forget about being a boring housewife or mother and it felt good to have people notice that I was looking nice. I felt like I had when I was single, except now I felt better. I really found myself looking forward to the attention, and the flirting a little. It was nice thinking I was still attractive after the years of being good, doing the shopping, washing, cooking, being as much with the children as I could, and trying to work. This put the feeling of being "worth something" back into me.

Patrick and I saw less and less of each other, as he would come home from a three-hour run, or an evening in the pub, and I would go out. We grew further and further apart, as well as the difference in interests, we finally even ran out of things to talk about. One particular day we had an argument about something, and both of us were angry. He was getting my chair out of the car and slamming the doors outside his sister's house, when he looked at me with a real distant look in his eyes of "I don't care" and saying, "Why don't you just go and meet someone else then, someone that will make you happy." With that I felt really angry and thought, "OK, if that's how you feel I will."

We left his sister's after a BBQ in the garden, and I was still upset and angry. Patrick could be stubborn as well as me, so we didn't speak again for the rest of the day. We got home and although I did not feel in the least like going out, I felt I would go anyway just to get out of his way, and to bloody well meet someone.

It was quite late so I decided to go straight down to the club rather than to a pub. I was sitting at the bar ordering a drink and standing next to me was someone I had not noticed in there before. I looked up and he was smiling at me. "Hello," he said with a big smile on his face showing a set of lovely teeth. Teeth and eyes are two things I always notice on a man, and both were very welcoming. I can remember the impact this man had on me, and even to this day still has.

He grinned as if he had known me forever, giving me his hand and introducing himself as Phillip. He was wearing a nice blue shirt, crisp and clean, blue jeans and his hair was slightly grey. Straight away I warmed to his manner and in fact I melted to him. He was very lively and full of fun, and we laughed and chatted for hours. After just a while I felt as if I had known him for a lifetime. He told me he had just gone through a nasty divorce and his two young sons were living with his ex-wife ten miles away. I explained my situation, in that I was married with two children, but not very happy in the relationship, and he understood. I wasn't even aware of the time, and when the club closed, we left together and talked outside. I told him I would get a taxi home. He lived just a couple of yards from the club and as I waited for the taxi he asked if I would like to go around to his flat tomorrow evening. I blurted out with excitement, "Yes I would." I knew it was wrong as I was married, and I should not put myself in that situation, but I don't think wild horses were going to stop me. I honestly believe it was love at first sight. He waved me off as the taxi took me up the road and his figure grew smaller and smaller as he disappeared into the distance.

That night I didn't sleep a wink, going over all the things we had talked about. I kept seeing his cheeky blue eyes and his lovely smile. I tried to concentrate and focus on my real life back home, my kids, Patrick, the lodgers, the students, I should be sensible.

The next day my poor mum was admitted into hospital, so my dad and I had a gruelling journey thirty miles away to see her. She had to stay in for a while. I kept saying to myself, should I go out tonight or not. My heart really wanted to see him again, but my sensible head was saying no. Dad and I left the hospital about six and we drove home quite fast as he had to get back, which made me pleased as I too wanted to get home as soon as possible. After such a bad day I kept telling myself it would be a reward for me to see Phillip. Was I just making excuses for what I really wanted, or was I justified in my actions?

I went home first to make sure the children were OK and got ready quickly. Patrick and I were still not talking so I kind of grunted as I went out of the door. I had arranged to go to my friend's house before ringing Phillip. She lived just up the road and opposite to his flat. I rang him as arranged and my heart was thumping so fast as I hadn't felt like this for years. He answered, sounding happy that I had remembered. I told him my friend would walk me down.

There were five steps to his flat, but my friend was used to getting up and down them as she had steps of her own. She dropped me at the door, I rang the bell and he welcomed me in. My mouth nearly fell to the floor, as he had such a nice flat, with good taste in colours. It was beautiful and brand new. He had picked such warm colours with matching furniture. There were arches through to the kitchen which had a black marble work top with white units underneath. I could tell he hadn't long moved in as there were still cardboard boxes here and there and empty places for furniture where he hadn't yet found anything he liked. He showed me around and I said, "Wow, you have a great place." He was a very modest man, and often when complimented would play it down.

We again started talking and laughing as if he was my best friend of old. The longer I spent with him the warmer I grew to him. He treated me with love and care, and was so interested in what I had to say. This had been one thing I had been desperately missing from my husband. He was so funny as well, and his favourite music was Dire Straits, and the Eurythmics. We sang along to this, him playing his air guitar, and me with my pretend microphone.

I didn't want to leave his company, but when I looked at the time it was 2 am, and the time had gone so fast. I had to go now or I wouldn't be able to get my taxi home. He offered to take me in his blue BMW which was parked outside his window, but I didn't feel it would be right, so I got the taxi instead. We arranged to see each other again the next night. I had told him where I lived and he said he had to drive past there every morning and evening on the way to and from work. He said he would look over and beep his horn at my house. I said I would look out of the window especially at 4.30 pm as I knew I would be home then doing the cooking.

The next day couldn't come quick enough and I was waiting by the window when I saw his BMW go past. He looked over at my house, slowed right down and blasted his horn. It was so funny and this went on for days. My biggest concern was that Patrick would come home early and notice this strange routine we had.

Eventually I started to spend more and more time with him, until in the end I was staying the night. I had to lie to my husband about where I was, although my friends would cover for me, saying I had been with them if he should ask. Things were still very strained between my husband and me. I was drifting further and further away, as if on a raft heading out to sea. The more I fell in love with Phillip, the more I felt distant from my home. I still deeply loved my children, and felt so guilty at times. I just fell deeper and deeper in love with Phillip. Nothing would stop me and I once spent three whole days and nights with him. We would go out in the car singing and being totally happy, or we would be in bed having the most amazing sex ever. He didn't have any inhibitions and I never tired of his love.

The reality did hit home to him that I was in fact married, and it used to bother him, in fact he hated it. Many nights he would tell me that he loved me but said, "I hate doing this, it's wrong." He had been hurt in his marriage and didn't want to hurt someone else.

For me it was too late, I couldn't just give him up. Night after night I would rack my brain on what I should do. How could I get around this dilemma? So many times I thought if I left my marriage I could be with him. Then I thought about my children and couldn't do it. The other problem was he hadn't actually asked me to do that. He wouldn't have because if he had, it would have been breaking up the one thing he felt strongly about, not hurting anyone else. We were in one hell of a mess, so I had an idea. If I told Phillip that I had left my husband on my own accord, he would feel happier seeing me. So that is what I did. I lied through my teeth telling him I was living up the road now with my friend. "There," I thought, "that's all sorted for the time being." I was now lying to everyone including myself and this worked for a few months. I was juggling my life between the two worlds happy in the one with Phillip, and feeling guilty and miserable in the real one at home.

All this had to eventually come to a head. Many times my husband would question where I had been, even leaving me a note one morning saying, "I know you are seeing someone."

"Oh god," I thought. "What will happen if it all comes out?" He was good at burying his head in the sand, so I thought he would do it again and he did. Then the worst thing happened. Phillip was passing my house one day and saw me there. Now he knew that I had lied to him.

That evening he wouldn't answer the phone, so I got one of my friends to push me to his flat and I told her to leave me on the top of the steps. I knocked and he wouldn't answer, yet I knew he was in, as his car was outside. He was ignoring me and I started to get frantic, I had to speak to him to explain. I knocked harder and started shouting and begging him, "Please open the door and let me in." A few minutes later he reluctantly opened the door to me. I was crying so hard I could hardly speak. I sat on the settee, where so many times we had made love, and he sat as far away as he could. I begged him to cuddle me. "Please cuddle me," I sobbed. He got up and brought me some tissues and asked if I wanted some tea. He then went on to say it was over. I didn't blame him at all, as I was stupid for trying to keep him by telling lies. It was just a matter of time. The one thing I could not understand was that he then asked if I would stay the night. I said no and left.

My life was never quite the same after that and I felt so desperately sad without him. He had been my world and now he was gone. My children would chat away to me saying "Mummy, Mummy," and I would be on autopilot with the answers. I hoped that they couldn't see the sadness in my face. I just carried on as if nothing was wrong and I was driving my close friends crazy, as they were the only people I could talk to about it. Patrick didn't say any more about the note, and neither did I. I carried on going out in the evenings, and in some ways that made it even harder, as I missed Phillip so much. I would still see him out with his friends sometimes, he was never nasty or rude, and would often ask me if I was OK. I would put on a brave face and say "Yes."

I did have one very weak moment a few days later however. I was in a room full of people, feeling so alone. Everyone seemed to be laughing and happy. I thought, "What is there to be happy about?" I looked over at the phone in the corner, and the next thing I found myself dialling his number. His voice came down the phone, bringing back all the feelings I had for him. Hearing him I wasn't sure if I should say something or put it down. I then found myself saying, "Phillip it's me, please can I just meet you and talk?"

He replied, "I'll come and get you."

The next thing he was pushing me up the road just like the old days. We went into his flat, and he said, "I'm just building some wardrobes." We went into the bedroom where there were bits everywhere and I sat on the floor watching him as he screwed it together. We just talked normally, nothing heavy or about us, just general chat. Then his phone rang and it was work. He said, "I have to go out," and I asked if he would mind dropping me back down the road. We said goodbye and I went home feeling a little bit happier, but knowing we could not carry on as it was over, and I had to accept it. A few months later I heard he was seeing someone else, and later he got married to her and moved to New Zealand.

Chapter 14
The Fire

Things were still the same at home regarding Patrick and I, although we both carried on being there for the children, who were now both at school and doing well. I was still working for the taxi company and taking in students. I remember the day our house caught fire as this was a terrible experience for me.

I had been on the beach in the afternoon and was deciding if I should go straight to work or go home first. In the end I decided to go home and get ready, as I had a long night ahead of me.

I was in the bathroom washing my face, when suddenly I heard an almighty bang from behind me. Opening the door of the airing cupboard where the immersion heater was fitted, I was greeted by a huge flame and loads of smoke. I knew I had to shut the door immediately to keep the fire in, and get out of the house as quickly as possible. The electricity had all gone off and therefore my stair lift was not working. I managed to climb/crawl down the stairs as quickly as possible. In fact I ended up almost throwing myself from top to bottom, as the smoke was following me down. I had a second wheelchair at the bottom and I climbed into this as fast as possible. I then quickly pushed myself into the living room where there was a phone. I dialled 999 and told them what had happened, also explaining that I was in a wheelchair. They asked if I was alright and I said "Yes" and told them I thought I would be able to get outside by myself. As I looked around the smoke was now completely everywhere and I was finding it hard to breathe. Reaching the back door, as it was my only ramped access, I managed to get out and wait on the drive. As I looked up my heart was in my mouth, as smoke was now belching from every single opening possible. I didn't panic, even though seeing the smoke coming out of the roof and every window was such an awful experience.

Soon I heard a siren. "Good," I thought. "Help is here." Unfortunately it was just a police car. He seemed to be in more of a panic than me, and I remember him asking where the source of the fire was. I told him it was in the airing cupboard upstairs. He tried to open the back door (which I had closed on the way out) and the smoke billowed out and stopped him in his tracks. Then I heard another siren and another, until three fire engines were now parked up outside and firemen were running everywhere with breathing apparatus, hoses, the lot.

Then it started to sink in that my home was about to be destroyed, along with all our belongings. The next car to pull up was Patrick and the kids, which he had just collected from school. He told me that as he was driving up our road, he could see all these fire engines and as he got closer and closer, he couldn't believe it was actually our house. One of our neighbours had kindly offered to take me and the children in, as I was by now shaking uncontrollably. She handed me a cup of tea, and I remember shaking the cup which kept hitting the saucer. "Sorry," I apologised. I was scared I would break the cup, as it was hitting the saucer so hard. My mouth was dry, I couldn't stop crying, and as I looked down at my children, cuddling them, I kept thinking, "What if they had been in the house, what if it had happened in the night, we could have all been killed."

The fireman eventually put the fire out and in the process they had taken out the whole landing window frame at the top of the stairs. They had to do this to throw out all the stuff that had been on fire in the airing cupboard. The whole lot was in the rear garden, blackened and burnt, every towel, sheet and bit of bedding was gone. The house was full of black smoke and water, not one room was saved. The worst thing was that we didn't have any house insurance. The property inspector came out and checked to see if it was still safe to live in. It was, but the clean-up process and the awful smell went on for weeks and weeks.

Mentally I found it hard also as I kept thinking if it could happen then it could happen again, perhaps when we were asleep. I kept thinking is the light switch safe or are all the appliances unplugged at night? It took months before I settled down and accepted it was a one-off faulty switch in the airing cupboard which should have been replaced a long time ago, but slipped through the net. That day we were supposed to be taking on two new students, but all that had to be cancelled. The council did give us a cheque for the towels and the bedding, which they didn't have to, but it was very difficult and took us a long time to get over this event.

Chapter 15
The Break Up

Months passed by, and Patrick and I had virtually been living two separate lives in one house. We were barely spending any time together, he not caring if I was in or out and I doing likewise. Our two worlds were so far apart, and I found myself spending more and more time with my friends and work colleagues. I was happy in my own little world I suppose, although on looking back I think I was desperately looking for someone to care for me. I needed someone that wanted to be with me and love me, not just put up with me, or be there for the sake of our children. They were doing well at school and I think Patrick and I did a pretty good job of hiding our attitude towards each other in front of them. He was still being a wonderful dad to them, looking after them in the best way possible, and probably far better than me.

My life had spiralled a little out of control as I was going out most nights either alone or with my friends. One evening I remember, it was a Tuesday, I hadn't been feeling great in myself, and I had been considering all evening if I should go out. I had been lying on the settee when Patrick arrived home and since he wasn't in the best of moods that made me decide to go out. Before I knew it I was on the phone dialling a taxi. Whilst I waited, I brushed my hair, and put on a nice new pink top with a mohair cardigan to match. Looking in the mirror I hoped I looked better than I felt. The taxi arrived and because it was late I went straight to the local club. I found the usual friends in there to talk to. I was circulating round some, as I always hated spending all evening with just one person. I would go here and there to talk and laugh with everyone.

I was deep in conversation with a friend but couldn't help looking over to the bar area, and seeing a man looking over at me intently. His eyes were almost fixed on my every move. At first I tried to ignore him, but no matter how hard I tried I could feel these big brown eyes penetrating right through me as if he was so intent on getting my attention that nothing was going to stop him. I didn't like to be rude to anyone that ever smiled at me as I felt if they were kind enough to give a smile, I should be kind enough to accept it, and return the gesture, which I did. After a few more minutes I had broken off my conversation with my friend and found myself being drawn by this stranger to the bar. I said, "Hello," and he promptly replied in a very northern accent, "Hello, I'm Colin." He then went on to say how attractive I was, and despite being shy, he couldn't help but want to talk to me.

Colin had a young fresh-looking face, dark hair and big brown eyes. Straight away I got the impression he was not at all used to chatting up women. He came over as very humble, almost as though he felt he was intruding on me. I reassured him I was happy to meet him and I suggested we leave the bar area and go and sit at a table so we could talk properly. Colin was quiet in his manner, so being near the bar made it difficult to hear him as clearly as I wanted to. We found a nice table under an arched area of the club, it held just two tables and the other one was vacant, so we had the place to ourselves.

Colin told me he had come down here on holiday with his parents, he said he didn't want to come initially and it took a lot of persuading from them. He had just gone through a rather nasty divorce, and his parents thought it would do him good to get away for a holiday. It wasn't his idea of a grand time as his parents were happy to go to bed early, leaving Colin on his own in the evenings. He had been down on holiday for three days, OK in the day but bored to tears in the evenings. So on this particular night he had done something totally out of character for him. He had started talking to some men that had been working for British Petroleum. They asked if he wanted to join them in this club, but as he wasn't a member he didn't think he could get in. The men he had talked to told him not to worry, as they would sign him in even though they had only just met. So there he was in a club where he wasn't a member and talking to me. We stayed in deep conversion until the club closed.

I was listening to his story, how his wife had an affair and that he had a little boy of only two. I told him my story, my unhappiness at home, and about my two children who were now six and four. We got on so well and I was thinking to myself, "I actually believe everything he is telling me." Sometimes when I meet men and speak to them for the first time, I think to myself, "Pull the other one, it's got bells on." I have a lot of trouble trusting men, as so many would lie to you just to get you to have sex with them. Then you find out they are married or something. But with Colin I never for one moment disbelieved what he was telling me. I liked his gentle and polite manner. The club closed and we talked whilst I waited for my taxi to take me home. Colin asked if I would like to go out again tomorrow in the day. Quickly I thought about how I could do it, and before I knew it I had agreed to meet him at 2 pm the next day. I gave him my address, as I knew Patrick would be working, and the children would be at school. I remember thinking after how risky it was, what if Patrick didn't go to work or the children were ill and didn't attend school? It was too late and before I knew it I was heading for home in my taxi leaving Colin outside the club with my address in his hand. Then I thought perhaps he wouldn't turn up, but I knew I wanted to see him again as I had started to like him.

Morning came, and the usual routine went to plan, Patrick took the children to school and then went off to work. I got up and decided to give the house a good clean, just in case Colin did turn up.

It was just before 2 pm when I saw a light green Triumph Acclaim pull up outside. I looked through the curtains and looked into the car and saw that it was Colin, he had remembered, right on time as well. I opened the door with a smile as he got out of the car, and I could see he was as nervous as me. He looked clean and smart and leant over me giving me a hug. I invited him in but only for a minute, as I didn't feel it was right to stay in Patrick's house with another man. Shortly after we left, I got into his car and we started driving off.

"Where would you like to go?" he said, smiling over at me.

I replied, "I don't mind, but seeing as you probably don't know your way around here too well, shall I lead the way?" Colin was happy with that and I knew I had about four hours before I should be home. I suggested we go to another seaside town twenty miles away.

It was August, the perfect summer's day, sunshine and just a nice temperature. We talked so freely and I felt totally comfortable in Colin's company, and it felt almost as if I had known him forever. All the nerves had gone, the radio was playing and the warm summer breeze was sweeping through my hair, I felt at that moment as if I didn't have a care in the world. We arrived at the seaside town and went along the beach front. Since Colin came from a city he really appreciated the view. We ate ice cream and talked about our lives. The time just flew by and before we knew it, it was time for me to go back. We didn't stop chatting all the way home, he said he had told his parents all about me, and they had asked if they could meet up. Colin asked what I was doing this evening. I knew I wanted to see him again, that was for sure and I agreed to meet him again that same evening.

I arrived home by taxi from town, as I didn't want to be dropped off by Colin, as I knew people would be home by now. I did the usual things at home, cooked the tea for everyone, talked as normal, but my mind was in the clouds thinking about Colin. I got ready and went back out. No questions had been asked by Patrick as we had both stopped that a long time ago. Having total freedom meant I could come and go as I pleased.

I met Colin in a nice pub just off the main road near the sea front. He greeted me and then introduced me to his mum and dad. They seemed as friendly as him, strong northern accents with a good firm handshake from his dad and a kiss on the cheek from his mum. "Nice to meet you, love," they said. Colin had told them all about me, even my circumstances at home. I was worried about that, as they had just seen their son go through a divorce so I didn't think they would want him to get involved with a married woman. Even if I didn't act married I knew I still was.

They seemed fine chatting to me all evening, saying how they loved it down here by the sea. Colin had been telling me how he was a security guard in Sheffield, explaining the long hours he had been working, sometimes sixteen hours a day, with a long drive to and from work. He had sold his house and was now in a flat in Sheffield, which he was in the process of decorating. He said he had enjoyed his holiday here. I was growing to like Colin's personality more and more. He had such a lot of gentleness about him and seemed extremely caring toward me. In fact nothing was too much trouble for him, the wheelchair or pushing me, it all seemed so natural for him. I continued to see Colin every night he was down here on holiday and in between in the day time. When I wasn't able to meet him, he would ring me from a phone box. Saturday came and it was the day for Colin to go back to his hometown of Sheffield. I felt sad, as if I was going to lose my best friend.

The morning he was due to leave I woke up thinking I just had to meet up with him one last time before he went. I was like a woman possessed. It was tricky that day as Patrick and our family had arranged to go to his sister's in Wiltshire, about fifty miles away. I got up really early and got ready, thinking if I rang the hotel where Colin was staying he wouldn't mind meeting me for a few minutes. I had one problem, which was that Patrick had to do something early that morning and that meant I was left with my children. "I will just have to take them with me," I thought. I called the taxi company and they collected us, dropping us in town. We popped into a shop first as I wanted to buy Colin a present, just a little something that he could have to remember me by. I found him a mug which when you tipped it up it spoke to you. I found this funny and thought he would too. The hotel had got hold of Colin, so we arranged to meet outside a pub. My children asked what are we doing and I said we are just going to meet a friend. They seemed to accept this with no more questions.

We met at eleven, I gave him the present and he was so surprised that I had gone to so much trouble to meet him. My children sat quietly on the bench outside, sipping away on their orange juice and looking over their tall glasses at Colin. Colin and I had coffee and then as much as we were able to do in front of my children, said goodbye to each other, telling each other to take care and that we would speak on the phone. Then Colin walked off up the road with his gift in his hand, leaving me for what I thought was forever. I wanted to cry I felt so sad.

I kept wondering if he would really ring me, after he got back home or if he would just get on with his life in Sheffield. He had told me he had just started to see a Greek girl, but he wasn't sure if they were suited, as she had very different ideas on life than him. For instance she wanted to get married and have at least five children, whereas Colin couldn't think of anything worse. He had only been seeing her a few weeks and already had a lot of doubts. Still, in the back of my mind I had to accept he was going home and my life was here without him.

Patrick was ready and waiting for us when we got home. We set off for his sister's and I remember being quiet as I didn't really want to talk to anybody. I tried to act normal but all the time it was hard. I looked at my watch at two o'clock, wondering how far away Colin was now. The road to Patrick's sister's was very bendy and slow, it seemed to drag on forever, except in one way I didn't mind as that meant less time in front of everyone trying to act happy and normal, when all I really wanted to do was be alone. It was a nice sunny day again, the children had fallen asleep in the back of the car, and Patrick was concentrating on his driving with just the sound of the radio.

His sister had a big house with a massive garden for the children to play in, leaving the adults to talk in the house without being interrupted. Our two children and her two played happily together. Patrick and her partner left us as they headed off for a drink at the local pub. I felt a bit uncomfortable about this, as I was sure I had "Guilty" written all over my face. His sister didn't seem to notice and in fact started to pour her heart out to me, telling me how she and her partner were going through a bad time. I listened intently and sympathetically, saying yes and no in the right places. Part of me felt so sad for her, whilst the other part of me had my mind on Colin. I was so desperate to see if he had arrived back in Sheffield safely. I had the number on a piece of paper in my handbag. I even contemplated asking her if I could make a quick call, but I would have not been able to talk properly on the phone. Just as I was thinking this Patrick arrived back, and suggested we all go for a walk, as it was such a nice evening.

We headed off into the village. My mind kept drifting and I thought now we were out, I was no way going to get the chance to ring Colin, as I certainly wouldn't have asked his sister now, not with Patrick being back. Then just there on the corner, outside of some shops was a phone box. "Oh," I said to Patrick, making some excuse, "I have just got to ring my friend up," lying through my teeth. I managed to not only get Patrick to put me in the phone box, but he said, "Do you mind if I leave you a minute and go in that shop?"

I was so relieved and I dialled Colin's number as quick as I could. He answered, he was so pleased to have heard from me so soon, and he said he had not been able to stop thinking about me all through the journey home. I was so happy to hear this. Then the next few words that I heard came as such a surprise. Colin said he had spent some time round at his parents' house after they arrived back in Sheffield. He told them how he felt about me, how he wanted to be with me. Then he announced that he had rung the firm he worked for and quit his job. He was prepared to move down here the following Tuesday.

I could not believe it. "What will you do about working?" I said. He replied that he wasn't worried, and that he would find a job when he got here. I explained I was in a phone box, and said I would ring him again at the first opportunity I had.

Putting the phone down I felt such a relief after the way I had felt before I rang. Before I was not sure if I would ever hear from him again, and now he was telling me he wanted to be with me, even sacrificing his job and his life in Sheffield. I only had to wait three days and he was coming back down. The rest of my day at Patrick's sister's was a bit of a blur with so many different things to think about, and it looked as if my future was about to change yet again.

I rang Colin the next opportunity I had which was on the Sunday morning when Patrick was out. We were both so excited, and I said I would try and find him somewhere to live, even if it was just a room for now. I called a close friend who used to be my boss, who had a five bedroom house with some spare rooms. He offered to let Colin have a room for a few days until he could sort something out.

Tuesday morning Colin set off. He arrived in the early hours of the morning and spent a few hours asleep in his car. He had driven to a small ferry, which crossed the water to my town. The ferry had not started yet, as it was too early. Therefore he parked up and caught up on some sleep. I waited at home for the phone call from him telling me he had arrived. This came through just after 8.30 am and Patrick was already out taking the children to school. "Well I'm here," he said when he rang. I met him as soon as possible. I was still in shock, one that a man had actually kept to his word, and two that he had really meant how he felt about me.

Next it was time to find a job. I knew a bakery two miles away which had a little flat above it and I knew this was empty so we headed up there to ask the owner if he would rent it. The news was better than we expected, not only was the flat vacant but they also had a job going in the bakery below. So after a few days Colin moved into the bakery and started his new job out in the country, delivering bread and cakes to local homes and shops. So different to his previous job, although he had to be up early, it was worth it to be out in the middle of nowhere, just pure countryside and farms. No hustle and bustle of city life. The flat had a rather steep set of stairs, which didn't make it easy for me getting in and out, but Colin never minded carrying me. Once inside the flat I was able to get around without too many problems. It was old and needed work doing on it and long term

I could never have managed to live there, but it did us at the time.

Colin initially kept his flat on in Sheffield, as he had to go back and see his little boy as often as he could. Just before he met me he had booked a holiday on the Norfolk Broads with a couple of friends of his, a work colleague and his wife. Colin asked if there was anyway I could get away and go with him for the week. So I told more lies to Patrick and somehow managed to pull it off. Before I knew it I was sitting in the beautiful sunshine driving a boat down the Broads. That was such good fun, as I didn't need my legs for that. We had a great holiday and laughed so much I couldn't remember when I had felt so happy.

On our return I was questioned by Patrick, but managed to change the subject. As I have said before, he was always so good at burying his head in the sand, which on this occasion I was glad of. My routine of being at home was completely a sham. I did feel guilty, but was in love with Colin. So every moment possible I wanted to be with him. He showed me such a lot of love and care and nothing fazed him regarding what I looked like, or that I couldn't walk. He would even do exercises on my legs in the evening to help the circulation, as the doctor had told me previously that this was important.

I felt I could be completely myself with Colin, naughty, funny and above all else loved. On most days that I wasn't working I would go out in the van and keep him company whilst he delivered the bread and cakes. We would stop off at the top of the hills admiring the view, eating the cakes and laughing at the real locals. Some of them had not been out of the village in their entire life. They all loved seeing Colin as he dropped in with the bread. For some of them it was their only communication in a day. Colin always had time to say a kind word to them.

A few months had passed and a few times I had been spotted by people that recognised me as I was being carried into the bakery. News soon got back to Patrick. I was being asked more questions and telling more lies. At home it had got to the point where we weren't sleeping together. I would go home and get into bed with one of the children, so as not to wake Patrick. Things went from bad to worse. Patrick started to get angry, saying, "I know you are having an affair, why don't you just admit it."

This did scare me, as I knew what I was doing was wrong, but at the same time I hoped I could have the best of both worlds. Now it seemed as if the bubble was about to burst. At first I didn't admit it, then after a sequence of events I had no choice. It was a make or break decision. Patrick was prepared to give me a day to decide if I would stay with him or choose Colin. Colin and I went out that day and I remember being in such a state. I loved Colin and although I had only known him for a few months, somehow I felt that if I did choose him, he would love and care more than Patrick had in the seven years we had been together.

I returned home, to the room in darkness. Just a faint flickering coming from the television, Patrick was on the settee. "Well," he asked, "what have you decided?"

My heart sank as I looked at him. "I haven't," I replied. I didn't want to hurt anybody, I really didn't; I felt such a bad failure.

"Then I'll decide for you," Patrick answered. The next day he got up and went straight down to a solicitor and filed for divorce.

The decision was now made. I looked at my children, and I felt so sad, hoping they wouldn't hate me for what I had done. I loved them so much and didn't want this to affect their little lives. But that is impossible. In the real world divorce means a lot of bad feelings, lots of anger and hate. That is what happened next.

Patrick and I were stuck. I couldn't move out, as I had nowhere to go as it was impossible to live above the bakery with Colin. Plus I couldn't risk leaving my home without having the security of another home that I would be able to live and manage in with my disability. On the other hand I did not in any way want to make Patrick leave his home. Life was incredibly hard for all of us.

All sorts of people got involved apart from the usual solicitors. We had social workers and housing managers, all trying to find the best way around this very awkward and delicate matter.

Patrick wanted me out and rightly I think, since any marriage that is at the point that we were would be the same. But I had nowhere to go. Some officials said I should fight for my children and stay in the home. I completely disagreed, not because I didn't want my children, because I did, but why should I punish Patrick for something I had done? He had always been a good dad and I was not prepared to do this to him or them. Part of me thought perhaps they deserved a life with him rather than with me. What standard of example had I shown them?

Eventually the council found a two bedroom flat in the town for Colin and me. It was dirty and in need of decorating badly, but at least it meant freeing everyone of the pain we were all enduring. I remember the day we got the keys for the flat, and I looked around thinking what a terrible mess. So different from what I was about to leave behind. That night I sat at home with tears in my eyes as I looked around. I had in the few months before Patrick and I split up, had nearly every room decorated. Now I was leaving it all behind. I was pleased for the sake of my children, as they now had nice bedrooms to grow up in with the latest all in one beds that sat above wardrobes and drawers. They loved them and enjoyed climbing up the ladder to the top. That evening I did cry. Patrick was home but didn't make much comment, which was probably just as well. I had arranged to leave when they were all out. This way would make it less painful for everyone.

Sunday morning Patrick and the children had arranged to be out. I had told Patrick that I only wanted to take my stereo and my clothes, everything else was his and the children's. Shoving my clothes into a black bin liner was strange as usually I did this if it was going to Oxfam or the bin. Here I was now putting my entire life into a number of black bags.

The flat was cold and empty and we had nothing except each other. We went to a second hand shop and bought a bed and all the basic bits and pieces. Neither of us had very much money, but we managed and would buy little bits when we could. It made me appreciate things that before I had taken for granted.

The first room we decorated was the spare room and we

managed to find some bunk beds, which meant my children could come and stay. Patrick knew I would have them any time he liked, and this meant he was free to go off running if he wanted to. At first it was hard for me, as I had a lot of guilt inside me. My friends were putting pressure on me, saying how ill Patrick looked, and almost like they expected me to go back. Sometimes I would be in a shop and Patrick would walk past the window looking so sad. He had also lost a lot of weight, and again I felt that this was my fault. I too had a lot of problems with my health through all the stress of the divorce and I too lost about three stone. I wasn't big before, and now I felt I too was fading away.

Things did settle down a bit after a few months for all of us, and my children knew they would still see me on a regular basis. They realised I was still in their lives and most importantly that I did, and will always, love them. My parents tried to remain neutral throughout all this, and they were always there for me, but didn't interfere. They only wanted what was best for me.

Chapter 16
Marrying Colin

Colin and I had been living together for a year, we never argued and life was good. We had built up a routine and were always there for each other. The one thing I think Colin found hard about being with me was my past. He lived in fear that I would want to go back to Patrick, even though I didn't ever think about that. Also being in a small seaside town, he had to see a lot of my ex-boyfriends, which again meant nothing to me, but for him, it made him insecure.

One day Colin asked me to marry him. I kind of brushed it off as I had thought previously that I didn't ever want to do that again. Not because I didn't love Colin, but because I didn't feel it was necessary. He had me, we lived together, why should we get married? But Colin kept insisting he wanted to, that he loved me and wanted to prove it to the world. He asked me to give my life to him. Those words were very powerful and meant so much to me.

In the end I trusted him and eventually I accepted, and hoped it would make him feel happy and secure. We set a date of the 3rd of November 1990 in a local registry office. We didn't want to put anyone to any expense as we had both been married before. We saved enough to pay for the wedding and a small reception after for family and close friends. A friend of mine made a wonderful cake. That morning Patrick dropped our children off with a look of sadness on his face. I felt so torn, not wanting to hurt Patrick any more, even though we were now divorced. I think he still found it hard that I was marrying Colin. I had bought the children some lovely outfits and dressed them up ready. I wore a purple dress and hat etc. and Colin had placed some ribbons on the car. He was dressed smartly in his suit and tie, and off we went. We were married at 10.30 with all our family and friends watching. The day was wonderful and my parents took the children back to their house as Colin and I headed off to a hotel for the night. I was now Mrs M.

A few months later we were offered a brand new house that was in the process of being built a couple of miles away. We were so excited and every week we would go up to view how the building work was progressing. We knew it was a huge step for us to go from our rather not so nice flat to a brand new house. Although life had become good in our flat, we had made some friends and it was just five minutes from the town centre. Somehow we had become rather used to it. The neighbours were OK, although you could hear everything above us, but I even got used to that in a funny sort of way. We had now managed to buy most appliances for a home, decorated most of the rooms, but hadn't managed to buy a carpet. It was such a big flat we couldn't afford to carpet the whole place. Only the children's bedroom and the lounge were complete, and the rest we just managed.

The big day came when the house was ready. I had been over the moon, and to this day can't thank the people enough who helped to put us there. It was a semi-detached house with two large bedrooms, a kitchen/dining room and a big enough bathroom for me to manage in. We had a stairlift fitted with a wheelchair at the top and bottom. Our furniture seemed to fit exactly and that night we went to bed, all snug thinking how lucky we were to have this new house. I couldn't sleep as there was something strange and I wasn't sure if I was imagining it or just being silly. Colin was also awake so I said, "Colin, I don't know about you, but I feel kind of lonely in this house." It was strange, knowing that there was no one above us or at the sides. No noise, just a complete silence. It took a little while to get used to, as for so long we had been surrounded by other tenants.

In between these events Colin's parents had also moved down

from Sheffield, and Colin had given up his flat there completely. First his parents lived in a flat in the same town, which was nice as we could go and visit them regularly. Colin would often drop them in some bread and cakes when he was doing his bakery round. I was still working for the taxi office part time and doing some voluntary work at our local hospital on the reception desk. Then apparently the contract on their flat ran out, so they decided to move ten miles away to a flat above a shop. I don't think his dad could really settle down here in the south, he would often unfavourably compare life down here with life back in Sheffield. He would often mention the cost of living being so much more expensive in the south of England. He had moved so many times in his life that he didn't really think too much of it, in fact when Colin was young he had attended sixteen different schools.

One evening Colin did the ten-mile trip to see his parents while I remained at home. When he came home he seemed different. I asked what was wrong and he said his parents wanted to move back to Sheffield. I was shocked but I guess not surprised as they had not been happy for a while. However what came next really knocked me for six. Colin announced he wanted to move back also, as he didn't want to live down here without them.

I was totally stunned. "When?" I asked.

"Within the next couple of weeks," he replied.

"But what about our house, my children, everything?" I started saying in a panic.

Colin said that although he loved me, he felt insecure here and needed to move back with or without me. We never really argued much before this event, but I remember getting really angry, as I didn't understand. He was the one that begged me to marry him. He was the one that said "Give your life to me." Now that I had done exactly that, I had "given my life to him" and he seemed to be throwing it back in my face, which was one thing I never thought he would do. Not my Colin.

"Please, why are you doing this?" I begged him. But there was no changing his mind. In fact the following week the three of them set off for Sheffield in a van, and I didn't even know if he was coming back.

I really thought I was going to die without him. I couldn't eat, my stomach kept churning over and I couldn't sleep. At the same time my one best friend in the entire world had just got married and was leaving our town to go and live in Wales. What a bombshell, and it felt too much for me to cope with.

I could not lose my Colin, I thought, I had to try, and as hard as I found it I tried living in Sheffield. He had rented a flat with stairs, which was very difficult. We had no money as we were paying for two properties, both north and south. I did try so hard, but we kept arguing as I resented him for breaking his commitment. I would feel really frustrated as I know things were hard for him but this was a bloody nightmare for me. My children were confused, as they had been used to me living just up the road. My daughter would write me notes saying, "We miss you mummy please come home." I would try to spend two weeks there and then come home. Sometimes Colin would come with me but often not. I had to rely on a friend to collect me from the train station, which was twenty miles from my home town.

On one occasion I was doing the Sheffield trip alone, when a man joined me and pestered me all the way to Birmingham. In fact he then tried to drag me off the train. Later I found out he had been out on bail so I think I had a lucky escape. It also taught me I should not be so friendly to people. After that train journey, I always kept my head down and didn't even smile at people.

This life of living in two places went on for a long time. I wasn't really sure where my home was anymore, and sometimes if I had been shopping, I was not sure if it was for here or in Sheffield. I did not feel I belonged anywhere.

One day his dad and I fell out, over me having a migraine. His dad really had it in for me, he was accusing me of many things, and when I tried to defend myself, Colin blamed me and said we were leaving. He marched me out of the door as though I was in the wrong. He didn't speak to me all the way down the long road back to the flat. I was crying but he took no notice. I said drop me at the train station as I am going home. Colin's dad and I didn't speak to each other for four years after that. He is very set in his ways. I was so cross at Colin that day, I had stopped at a phone box, and I remember ringing up my dad crying my eyes out, telling him what had happened. I told him how Colin had completely taken his dad's side, even though I hadn't done anything wrong. Being two hundred and fifty miles away my dad felt helpless and angry at Colin for doing this to me. Colin was always scared of his dad. He waited outside the phone box, said nothing and then dropped me off at the train station.

After I got home and had had time to reflect on what had happened, I wrote his dad a letter telling him how hard it was for me up there. I was wheelchair-bound in a city where I had no friends and in fact they were the only people I knew. I also reminded Colin that he should be looking after his wife, and that when you marry someone your priority should be your wife. Although you should be there for your parents as much as possible, your wife and your family should come first. The letter was discarded by his dad, leaving us not speaking for four years.

The double life, north and south, went on for about two years. Eventually I had had enough of all the travelling and insecurities that came from this division of two hundred and fifty miles. I said to Colin, "I can't keep this up. I'm going to go home and stay home this time. If you want me then you'll have to decide what you're going to do, and where you want to live."

Not long after that Colin did decide to come back and live with me in the south. We settled down and put the past behind us as much as possible. There was just one more occasion when things got on top of him. We had fallen out and I had gone to town with my friend. When I got home Colin had packed his things and left me and he had even taken the TV. He drove as far as Watford Gap and then rang me up to say sorry and came home. This was a delicate subject for me as Patrick had also done this before, and therefore I did find it difficult to get over.

Chapter 17
Children

Over the years the children came on in leaps and bounds. Colin's son would come down when he could and stay for a few weeks. My two were staying with us twice a week on a regular basis and were doing very well at school. Patrick, my ex-husband, had four years later remarried again. My children didn't really get on too well with his new wife, and so this created other problems. She had three children of her own, and five altogether must be a nightmare for any parent. I was always there for mine and did see them become increasingly unhappy at times. It was such a shame, as I think life with just Patrick by himself were the best years for them. They were so close, and he enjoyed looking after all their needs, so when he remarried, he too had to juggle on whom he should put first.

On collecting my son from school one day, he announced, "Mum, I'm not going home. I want to live with you." Now this was not a problem for me, but I was worried about Patrick, and how on earth he would take it. I told my son we would have to ring dad and talk it through, as it wasn't just my decision. Patrick came around and was devastated. I left them both to talk it through, and said I would go along with whatever decision they made. I didn't want to step on Patrick's toes, but at the same time I didn't want to reject my son, as I had always told them they had a home with me if they needed it. I remember sitting out in the garden looking at the flowers and playing with our dog while I waited. An hour or so later they both came out with red eyes where they had been crying. "Well, what have you decided?" I said. Patrick announced that they would be going home together. I accepted the decision and still tried to be there for my son as much as possible.

Next we had exactly the same thing from Colin's son when he came down to say with us. He said he wanted to live with us, and go to school with my two. There is one year between his son and mine, and three between his son and my daughter. Again we went along with it. His mother went berserk over the telephone when he told her. In the end they had to bribe him home by decorating his bedroom and buying him a puppy, and because of this he did go home at the end of the two-week holiday.

Finally it was my daughter's turn to have problems at the age of fourteen. She was having horrendous problems with her stepmother. Even a close friend of my daughter was concerned, as she had been staying with them. She was hearing and seeing things going on in the house and could see how upset my daughter had become. She asked if I was aware of these problems and I told her that I was, but again I didn't want to upset Patrick. The trouble was, Patrick was still burying his head in the sand. This time it was to the detriment of his daughter. Enough was enough, I thought, and this time I did not want people to stop her doing what she wanted. I figured she was now old enough to decide for herself. She said that she wanted to live with Colin and me and so that evening she packed her things and moved out from her dad's house. He was in a terrible state at the time, and I am sure to this day he will blame me. However my daughter did remain with us despite the stress of upsetting her father.

Colin and I over the years grew closer in a different way and we became the best of friends. He became so easy going, and far less possessive than in the earlier days. I think in the beginning he would always worry that I would want to go back to Patrick. As time passed into years, things became a lot more stable for us. He understood me in so many ways. I struggled in a lot of things, particularly with friends letting me down. Sometimes friends would be so hurtful by arranging events and not including me. I began to realise I didn't want to live in this small town any more, where everyone knew you and you knew everyone. I needed more in my life and felt I had a lot more to give.

Chapter 18
Hospital

My next two big goals were to try and find somewhere else to live in a much bigger town twenty miles away. We were there a lot anyway, as this was where the main shops were. So at least once a week we would travel there to do the food shopping. I liked this town and also the main hospital was here. There was a small hospital in my home town, but for anything major you would need to attend the main one.

My other goal was to try and get a job. I hadn't worked for a long time, even the bit of part time work at the taxi office had disappeared as the offices had merged with another company, giving them ample staff.

My dream was always to look after people. I had been attending an outpatient appointment one day and I noticed a poster on the wall asking for voluntary helpers. I jotted down the number, all excited, and wondering if they would accept me, being in a wheelchair. I contacted them straight way. I had to fill in some forms and I was accepted and was assigned a little post in Out-patients. However I found it frustrating, as I wanted to do more, but being voluntary there were a lot of issues with patient confidentiality. I persisted patiently and work followed in x-ray, Pharmacy and a couple of other wards. Eventually I was becoming well known to most of the hospital.

After a few months, I couldn't stand the frustration of not being more involved and I made some enquiries to see how I could apply for a proper job. I worked out that the best thing to do, would be to apply to go on the hospital job bank. I completed my forms and submitted them. The lady I had to see was very helpful and understanding. She understood my limitations, but at the same time wanted to give me a chance. A couple of weeks later she rang me at home asking if I thought I could be a ward clerk on the cancer unit. It was just going to be for a few weeks, as the woman who was currently in charge had been put on sick leave. I accepted the post even though I had never done this job before. I thought, "Well I have a challenge, and I am not going to be beat." I had common sense, and would do my best to learn the job. I went in a couple of mornings without pay, to see how the other lady managed. She showed me the ropes and I wrote down as much as I could.

I started the following week and now it was all down to me. I was nervous but did my best, although at times I felt like I was pulling my hair out. Not having a clue and with the ward very busy, I found that there were so many things to learn. After the first three weeks I finally felt as if I was getting to grips with it. My confidence was improving day by day and I really started to love it. I was only supposed to be doing it for three weeks, which in the end turned into six. I finished just before Christmas and the ward had even invited me to the Christmas party. I had made many new friends and was so sad it was all over. This meant going back to just doing my voluntary work again. It wasn't the money I wanted, it was the responsibility. I had had a taste of it now and I wanted more.

There was a job advertised for a ward clerk on another ward and I pondered over and over, should I go for this? It was full time, and I wasn't sure if I could do full time, as I hadn't worked for so long. Would the hours be too much for me? I decided to apply anyway and see how it went. I applied and got an interview. I found out the afternoon of the interview that I had been offered the job and I was delighted. I had been accepted and all my hard work had not been in vain. Now I would have my own ward to take care of.

I started my new post on the 4th of January. The whole ward was new, starting from scratch. New nurses were required and equipment was ordered. I had to learn my new job and fast. I had to hit the road running. The managers had agreed my hours at the time of interview. I would start off working full time, and see how I coped. I was happy about this, knowing that if I found it too much, I could reduce them to part time, and maybe job share. Every few months we talked to see how I was coping. Sometimes I found it hard as I was getting up at 6 am, being driven the twenty mile trip to work, then being collected after work and getting home about 6 pm. This was a very long day for me, especially with all the mental exhaustion from running the ward.

After a few months I heard there were some rooms available in a block of nurses' homes within the hospital grounds. I had tried desperately to move nearer in the last year or so, but nothing was happening. We had put our names in the paper for a house swap, and I had written to and rung the local council on a daily basis. I was now becoming desperate to move. Now I had a job, I had even more reason not to want to live here in my small seaside town, but move to where the hospital was. Colin and my daughter were very understanding about me wanting to work, and supported my decision. The mileage was taking its toll on the car, so I enquired about the rooms in the nurses' home, wondering if it might be easier to stay there Monday to Friday. They had a ground floor room available, which I took immediately, until we could find somewhere for all of us to live.

This arrangement worked a lot better and I didn't find the day so hard. At weekends I would go home. I had also built up a wide circle of friends from all departments.

Life was good, and I was happy, feeling needed in my job. Home life was stable and I knew that Colin wanted the best for me. He was so happy to see me working in this environment, as he knew it had been my lifelong ambition to work in a hospital rather than being a patient in one. He had become very close to my dad and the two of them would go out fishing together. My daughter had grown up a lot and she had a boyfriend and seemed happy too. I kept persisting with trying to find another place for us to live, and after four years of trying we finally found someone who wanted to swap. It meant leaving a bigger house to go to a small bungalow, but this didn't matter. My daughter had decided she wanted to move out and live with some friends and I was OK with this as long as she was happy.

Colin and I moved alone into the bungalow, which is just about a mile from the hospital. I kept my room on at the nurses' home initially until we had settled in and also in case my daughter wanted to move in there. In fact she did after a few weeks as she also went on to get a job in the hospital and therefore took over my room in the nurses' home.

The bungalow was a mess and needed a lot of work doing on it, but we didn't mind, as we were where we wanted to be. How nice it was to be away from that small seaside town. I didn't know many people in this new town, only the ones I had met through the hospital, and the best thing was they didn't know me either.

I spent several years working at the hospital, overseeing many changes. My boss who originally employed me had left. So many things were happening and changing at work, and not all for the better. My health wasn't as good as it should have been, and I didn't feel I had the same understanding from my new boss as I had from the previous one. Things were becoming harder for me. I had also decided after all the years of not singing that I wanted to try and start it up again. I felt that maybe I wanted to change my life, and I wanted to regain the chance I had been offered all those years previously.

I managed to reduce my hours to part time although this was quite a battle. When I wasn't working I would contact agents to see if they would be interested in my singing, or acting. I had never done acting before, but felt if I was given the chance I could do it. This worked and before long I had been accepted to do some plays. This involved working for a local theatre company. Before long I was touring schools and nursing homes. My role in this play was to open with a song I had written, then act and finally finish with another song. The next play was performed in the local theatre, and was about the Holocaust. It was fantastic and I had also managed to get myself on television, singing on a programme on Sky. I found out how to register with another television company and still remain on their database.

I love acting, but trying to fit in all the hard work that goes with it, the rehearsals and the travelling around, I found it was becoming impossible. Therefore after the last play finished I didn't return to do another one. I had to stay in my hospital job, as we needed the money. Acting was fun but unless I could be paid I wasn't able to continue. I had also applied for some singing competitions throughout the country and Colin would take me to these. It was all good fun and I often came third.

The final thing for me at the hospital came a few months later. I had some good news regarding my acting. Unfortunately I was not able to take it any further as the hospital wouldn't let me have the time off. So I decided I had enough and didn't want to work for someone else any more. I had made up my mind, and I came up with an idea that maybe there was a way for me to still look after people, but not from the hospital. I arranged to do a massaging course.

At first I was not accepted, because of the wheelchair. However I wasn't going to take this without trying first, so I pestered them continually until they let me on the course. I succeeded and passed. I then made the big decision to leave the hospital, and be brave and work for myself.

I registered self-employed as a market trader and holistic therapist. The market seemed another avenue. Our neighbour had been telling us how good it could be selling from this particular market and so eventually we decided to try it. One of the traders wanted out and offered to sell me a lot of jewellery, which I accepted. The market was Fridays, Saturdays and Sundays, and Colin would help me with this. The rest of the time I would concentrate on building up my massage business.

Chapter 19
Me as a Masseuse

Having now left the hospital, my whole world changed in a remarkable way. I had decided I still wanted to work with people to look after them and care for them, but I didn't want the responsibility I had had before at the hospital.

As a masseuse I would be able to work from home, do the hours I wanted, and be a free agent. I set about looking in the massage section of the paper to see how many women were doing this, wondering if I would be able to make enough money to make ends meet. Next I scanned the adverts to see if there were any massage tables, as I wanted to work from this rather than a bed, so as not to give people the wrong impression. I wanted it to look professional. I managed to find a nice second hand massage table in the paper for sixty pounds. I was pretty broke at the time and prayed I would at least be able to get enough money to pay for it. I then went on to put an advert in the local shops, again hoping I would be able to raise enough money to pay for the advertising. Next I bought a new phone so my number would be only for the people who wanted a massage, and not my personal one. Soon I was ready to go, adverts were in the shops, and my phone was connected. I was so excited and all I really needed was to wait for my certificate to arrive.

Within days the first phone call came through. I looked at the number and my heart was in my mouth, I was so scared. Suddenly I found myself answering, saying, "Good afternoon, can I help you?" A rather well spoken man on the other end was asking for details. I gulped and told him the price, which at the time was just £15 for half an hour. He seemed interested and I asked him to call tomorrow, as I was in town at the time and had to get back. However he said he would wait for me to go home if I didn't mind.

I rushed home as fast as I could, my head was spinning and my heart was racing. "Oh my God," I thought, "what if I'm rubbish? What if I'm not what he expected? What if I can't perform the massage to his liking? Well not on a real client anyway." This was different to just a few lessons on my course, for here I was faced with reality. I waited at the window, looking up the path. The massage table was all ready, with a nice clean towel in place. The oil was warmed, and my hands were shaking. I then saw a nice looking man walking up my path wearing a smart shirt and tie. He had dark hair and was of medium build. All sorts were running round my head and I blurted out, "Come on in," as I welcomed him into the lounge where the massage table was. He told me his name and shook my hand.

"What do you want me to do?" he said.

The truth was I didn't have a clue, but not wanting to sound as if he was my first I said in as much of a professional way as possible, "Would you like to remove your clothes, and just place them in the chair?" Then I remembered the consultation form and I handed it to him, asking him to fill it in.

As he removed his clothes I disappeared into the kitchen so as not to embarrass him. To be honest I was shocked as he removed all his clothes, including his pants. As I entered the room he was lying on his tummy showing his bare bottom. "Blimey," I thought, "I never expected that."

I was now faced with a naked man on my massage couch, and now I needed to impress and be confident so as not to show him I hadn't done this before. I asked him a few questions just to break the ice, and he was friendly and started telling me about a woman he was seeing at work. I sounded interested, but at the same time concentrating on how well I was performing the massage. I started on his head neck and shoulders, gliding the slippery oil all over his body, and I remember thinking what a nice body it was too. As I worked my way down, rubbing his legs, he started to part them a little so that I could rub my hand all the way up. He made a lot of good comments, saying "That feels good," and complimenting me on my techniques. After fifteen minutes, I asked him to turn over onto his back, so I could concentrate on the other side.

As he turned over I found it so embarrassing as I could see he had the hardest erection ever and this was something I hadn't bargained for. Over and over in my mind I kept wondering if I should say something or ignore it. But before long, he was asking me if I wouldn't mind wanking him off?

"Is this normal?" I said.

"Oh yes," he replied. "That is, if you don't mind." He said that all the other ladies he had been to did this, and they didn't mind.

Well before I knew it my hand and his prick were covered in oil, and I was wanking him off. I could see that his breathing became faster and faster, and then his chest rose suddenly and with a big explosion he emptied his hot spunk over his chest and my hand. "Thanks," he said, rising off the bed with a big smile on his face. I was just glad he was happy, and then I started to wonder what kind of road I was heading down. However I was now clutching the £20 note tight to my chest, as he had given me an extra fiver tip. I didn't really care. After all, I thought, I didn't have to do anything more than a hand job.

I didn't tell anyone, especially my husband, about what had happened, the reason being that he wasn't keen on me doing any of it to start with. We both knew we needed to earn more money, and weren't sure how, so this seemed to be an easy option. In my previous job I would have had to work nearly all day to get twenty pounds, whereas I had been given this for just half an hour.

My next few clients started coming in just from the adverts in the shops, and just like the first one, expected more than just their back rubbed. One man said to me, "If a woman don't do the hand relief, us blokes don't come back." That comment has always stuck in my mind to this day as I needed my clients to come back. I figured in this business you must create something that people enjoy, and I didn't really want to see one man and then never see him again. If that had been the case I would have seriously thought I was doing something terribly wrong.

After a few weeks I was starting to build up a regular few. One dear man named Nigel came to me one day. He never said a word all through the massage or hand relief. At the time I thought it was because he didn't like me, until he rang me the next day, and then the day after that, and so on for months. In fact he would see me nearly every night of the week. He was just shy to begin with. Nigel was a dear man, highly intelligent and had very white hair. Even though he was in his fifties, he looked a lot older. I grew closer and closer to Nigel over the months, until in the end I had to stop doing the massaging, as it didn't seem right. He had by now become a close friend to Colin and me. Sometimes on a cold winter's night when Nigel had been over, Colin would drive him the two-mile journey back to his house.

Nigel was a real genuine friend who would do anything to help me. He was always on the end of the phone and very often would buy me presents, or take us out for a meal. The one biggest thing with him was that he would sometimes lie, and I think looking back it was because he didn't feel he was good enough. So he would lie to make more of an impression. Nigel remained our close friend for two years until sadly he died of cancer very quickly. I miss him to this day.

A few weeks after starting the massaging my certificate came through saying I had passed. I was so relieved, as I had taken a big risk in giving up my hospital job, not knowing if I would be able to continue with the massaging. I breathed a sigh of relief as now I was officially a qualified therapist. In the meantime I had also taken on a market stall selling jewellery. Now there was no stopping me. I now had two businesses and although the market was hard going, with a lot of outgoings and often running at a loss, at least the massaging made up for it.

The next step was to find a better way of advertising, as the adverts in the shops were slow, with just a handful of calls a week. I checked out the local paper, and to my amazement there were about twenty other girls advertising, so I plucked up the courage and rang them, asking how to go about putting my ad in the paper. It was easy. They asked what I wanted to say and charged me accordingly. I didn't want it to sound seedy, as I was after all a qualified therapist. I tried to word it in a way that people would feel they were coming to someone that cared and to feel they could relax and unwind. Suddenly it all came to me, and what I should call my advert. "Relax and Unwind" with the rest including my phone number. They said it would go in tomorrow's paper.

The next day I didn't really think any more about my advert and I wasn't sure even what time the paper came out. I had had a slight headache around lunchtime and decided to have a lie down for an hour or so. I woke up after two hours, went into the front room and looked at my caller display. (This was just one of the safety measures I had put in place. I had also had an alarm fitted, CCTV cameras, number blocking and as much as I could do to keep myself safe.) The caller display said that I had missed ninety-nine calls in just an hour and a half. I was in total shock that one little advert had created such a demand. There had been about fifty messages too. I listened meticulously to each one, careful that if I was to make this business work I couldn't let anyone down. I thought if they were kind enough to ring, I should be kind enough to call them back if they had asked me to.

The next few weeks remained the same, I was always aware when I took a call that this might be a person who could have a bad intention towards me. There are a lot of strange people out there so I always went with my instinct. If I didn't like the sound of someone on the phone I just simply said, "I am so sorry I am busy," so as not to cause any problems. I think this worked and eventually they would give up trying.

One thing I found hard to understand at first was that all the calls were coming from men, even though I never stated in the advert that it was for just men only. I soon came to understand why. I met one man after another on a daily basis, and found to my shock, nearly all of them wanted more than just a massage.

Not all, but most would get very turned on during the massage. I wasn't sure if I should ignore this or what the rules were, for in those early days I was so ignorant. I remembered the first client I had had and the fact that I did give him hand relief although much to my shock at the time.

What was the golden rule here? Firstly when they arrived I suggested they pop their clothing in the chair before lying on the massage bed. I never ever said remove everything. Sometimes they would say, "Shall I take my pants off?" Getting used to being asked this question, I always replied the same. "I never ask people to do that, it's entirely up to you." Most would go for it and drop their pants as quick as saying "Jack Robinson". I tried to act as if I wasn't surprised so as not to embarrass them. I would put on some nice relaxing music, and set the lighting low. I had candles and pretty lights around, making it feel as warm and comfortable as possible. They would lie there on my massage table totally relaxed as I glided my warm slippery hand all over their body, and I would get such a warm feeling of achievement. They would make comments like "That feels so good", and this would boost my confidence even more. I thought I had found my vocation in life. Here I was, still looking after people but in a different way.

I soon came to realise that nearly every man that came to me did in actual fact want a complete – and I mean *complete* – body massage. I grew more confident in what I was doing, and in fact I had now built up a complete set routine. I would first start on their head, neck and shoulders, and then work my way down their back, pouring nice warm oil onto their buttocks and caressing them. Then slowly and very gently with the tips of my fingers I would tease just inside their thighs and touch their balls. After this I would turn them over onto their back. It was evident that they were aroused as their cock would be standing up like the Eiffel Tower. It would be so big and hard, just waiting for relief from my magic hands. I had a standing joke with my regulars that the face hole on the massage table was in the wrong place. By now it was clear, from the physical evidence and their comments, that they wanted me to wank them off. My hand would glide down onto their hard cock, using different techniques depending on how turned on they were. I didn't want it to be over too soon, so I learnt over the course of time so many ways to wank a cock. I never had a complaint, and was told by all of them how good I was. The more I did the better I became, learning different things from different men. Some liked it hard, others liked it soft. In the end it was second nature to me and I swear I have grown to know more about men's bodies in the last few years than they knew about themselves.

My regulars were building up more and more, which was nice as the nerves would sometimes be hard to cope with when I saw a new one. It was a bit like a blind date, not knowing who was going to walk in the door. Lots of thoughts would run through my head. What if they didn't like me, especially as I was in a wheelchair? But it became clear that most people were fine about it, and once I settled them onto the couch and worked my magic hands on them, they completely ignored the wheelchair. The proof that I was doing something right was when afterwards, just a few days later, they would ring me and ask if they could come back. I was delighted and most of them have been coming to me for five years now. I thank you to this day.

One of the downsides to this job was that some men are never grateful to just be given hand relief. Time and time again, I would be asked to do more. I would politely reply, "No, sorry, I just do massage with relief." Some would accept that and respect my service, and some would pester and pester me over and over, still trying to touch me. I hated it when men would try to put their hands on my legs or lift my skirt. I felt this was a real invasion of my right to say no. I would take their hand away, while trying not to upset them or make them angry, otherwise it could have turned nasty and I certainly didn't want that. I would make a little kind of comment like "That's naughty" as I removed their hand from my skirt.

At first I wouldn't let them touch any of me. But after time I accepted it wouldn't hurt if they just played with my tits. If that kept them happy, and made them come easier without wanting to go any further, then I was prepared to let them. Often I would enjoy it if they touched me gently. I have very sensitive nipples and love having them played with, so this did give me a lot of job satisfaction. After all, you have to have some perks of the job!

I grew to like my job more and more, making some good friends who I found to be there for me. I kept to my policy, even though some of my clients were rather persuasive by offering me more money, and trying harder to make me give in. I kept telling myself it was a very thin line between what I was doing, and what they wanted me to do, which was full sexual intercourse. At times it was hard but my conscience kept telling me to say no, stay as you are. I had just enough money coming in to pay the bills by charging for my massage service only. However there was never enough left over for treats, as I had built up a lot of debt over the last few years. Looking back I feel I tried to escape from the real world I was living in and I would run up store card and credit card debts. At the time it would make me happy by being able to have something I wanted by just handing over a card. However reality would sink in when the bill dropped on the mat. I was soon in a no-win situation. I had to do the job, just to keep the amount I needed keep coming in. No way could I go back to a normal job earning five or six pounds an hour. The debts had escalated out of control. I was trapped in this situation and I had to continue just to survive; this was hard.

I had some clients that I warmed to more than others, and sometimes they would stop and chat for long over their time. I didn't mind as I knew if I had another call come in they would go straight away, respecting that I had to take bookings.

My first special friend was called Stuart. We were chatting one day, and he mentioned a site on the internet, a site where clients could post ratings about the girls they had seen. Basically telling other punters the truth about girls rather than the girls telling things about themselves which might or might not be the truth. Stuart always said how good I was at my job and asked if he could put a recommendation on this site telling people about me. I agreed, as I trusted him even though I wasn't at that time very computer literate. I did say to him, "Please only put the truth, and also tell them I don't offer a full personal service." I had learnt a lot of the lingo spoken in terms of my job. The first time I was asked if I did a full personal service I ignorantly asked what is that. The poor bloke must have laughed his socks off at my ignorance. Still now I had been doing this for a few months I had learnt the abbreviations and meaning of most things I was asked for.

I had asked Stuart to put in another number for the recommendation, as I wanted to know where men had seen or read about me. A few days later the mobile number I had given Stuart was going crazy. Calls were coming in faster than I could cope. They were saying, "We've read such nice things about you. When are you available?"

Curiosity got the better of me. What had been written about me for so many people to call? I texted Stuart and asked him the name of the site, as I had not remembered it at the time. I looked it up through Google and there I was. I gulped as I was on a site that was advertising prostitutes. Oh my god, I thought, what have I done? There I was for the entire world to read. The one good thing was that at least he had said I did not offer a full personal service. He had complimented me, by telling people what a good service I offered, describing also that I was in a wheelchair. This was good as at least I knew when people rang me, they were fully aware of my disability. The phone was red hot and not one person seemed disappointed in me or disputed what had been written. Often men would go away and leave another report on the site. This all helped me and this also meant less advertising in the local paper. In the first year I had spent over £4,000 on adverts. It was the best thing Stuart could have done for me, and I thank him to this day.

So now I was getting regular clients from the local paper and the internet. My confidence was growing daily and it seemed that each man I met taught me something different. One of the first clients had asked me if I would just very gently, with the tips of my fingers, stroke his legs after he had climaxed. He said it was an amazing feeling, and it helped him to totally relax. I wondered if this technique would work on other men. I soon found out it most certainly did. Then I tried using different strokes during the massage, and I had hit on something really big here. I found out the most sensitive areas on men's bodies and now I had something to work on.

I would still feel extremely nervous when the phone rang, and it was a new one. I didn't tell the men who rang from the advert in the paper that I was in a wheelchair, as I thought this would put them off before they had even given me a chance. I would wait on the other side of the massage table for them to walk in. My first reaction was important and I thought I must act confident. This worked and I would make them feel at ease by asking what sort of day they had, and asking them to pop their clothes on the chair. Generally being nice to them from the start was a bonus. All I had to do now was put my hands on their bodies, and let my hands do the talking for me. Again I found this to be a gift I had.

Before long I had been given a name by my clients: "Magic Hands". They said this as they lay there moaning with ecstasy as my hands did the business for me. After about ten minutes they would totally relax, forget I couldn't even walk, and enjoy the time they had booked.

I felt almost as if I had found my vocation in life. I grew closer and closer to understanding men, what their needs were, and even how they needed as much attention as women do. I was almost an agony aunt to most of them. They felt as if they could come to me not only to satisfy their sexual desire and get the relief from climaxing, but they could also talk to me about all their problems. Sometimes they would have major issues at home, where their wife or partner didn't understand what they needed.

I began to realise that women were making big mistakes regarding their men. It was as if they were totally unaware of their partners' physical needs. Most men would tell me their partner had not been interested in sex for a very long time. It was as if they could just ignore the fundamental fact that their men had strong sexual desires and this in turn would then lead to men fantasising about going elsewhere. Not that they wanted an affair, as a lot of men I spoke to said they didn't want this. They said they still loved their wives, but couldn't manage with very little or no physical contact. I would often suggest that they talk to their partners, but even with them trying that, the women were totally blind to their men's needs. This would then lead them to come and visit masseuses like me. I think sometimes men need to have something to look forward to, and to be pampered just like a woman.

Chapter 20
Strange Requests

I have had some very funny and extraordinary requests whilst I have been doing the massaging. One day the phone rang and it was a man asking if I would be prepared to tie him up. I tried to explain that I do massaging, not bondage. He kept ringing and ringing begging me: "Please," he said, he told me he wanted to be tied up and left in a room for a few hours. He suggested I tie him up and either go out leaving him there, or tie him up and carry on working in the other room, but just keep coming in and teasing him every so often. In the end I had to tell him I was in a wheelchair as this was a man ringing me from the advert in the paper. He said he didn't mind and I then went on to explain that I would not be prepared to tie him up and leave him for hours in case something happened to him. Also I was worried that if I went out he would break free and burgle my home, and he did understand this. Weeks went by and he was still ringing me, begging me to just tie him up on my massage table and tease him. After many weekly phone calls I started to give in. I told him the price for an hour and he agreed. I then said I didn't have any gear to do this sort of thing.

He said without hesitation, "Oh don't worry I have the lot."

"The lot?" I thought. "Whatever does that mean?" I was soon to find out.

The next day he arrived at my place with two bags full of gear. Spreading it all out on the massage table, he explained to me where all the ropes, chains, belts and other things were to be applied. I had never seen such items before in my life and I started to feel very uneasy at this point, wondering what I had let myself in for. So many questions and worries were running through my head. What if I tied him up and something happened to him? Worried, I asked him what I should do next. He then proceeded to pull out of a bag a black PVC outfit that looked like something Spider Man would wear. He climbed into it as I watched in horror, trying desperately not to laugh. The outfit covered his head, leaving his face open, with another opening for his cock and balls. He started to get very excited by now, telling me where and how to use the rest of the gear. I tried to pull myself together and thought, "Well he seems to know what he wants," and I went along with his requests

"Tie my hands there with those leather straps," he said and then proceeded to give instructions about his legs. He placed himself onto the massage couch, lying flat on his back. He handed me the chains and ropes, and asked me to tie them to the massage table. I did as instructed. Lastly he said, "You have to stick this ball in my mouth and gag me."

"Oh my God," I thought, "he won't even be able to speak." Before I did this I asked him, "How will I know if you want to get out if you can't talk?"

He said, "Don't worry, I'll make you aware with my hand," which of course was tied by now to the massage table, leaving only his fingers free to wiggle.

I had done as instructed to the last detail, even pulling his head down really tight onto the massage table with some big leather straps. Next I was told to just leave him there. I had been instructed beforehand to tease his cock, which was standing up through the gap in the PVC suit as hard as rock. I kept flicking it with my fingers. I could see how aroused he was getting as a little bit of spunk was just leaking out of the end of his hard throbbing cock. I didn't want to make him shoot his load too quick, so I would get him to the brink, and then leave the room for a few moments, keeping an eye on him from the kitchen. I was also told to use strict words of punishment. I did this and I told him what a naughty boy he was and that he deserved to be punished in this way. I spoke in a very strict and meaningful voice, almost as if I had been doing this for years. I had lost my nerve by now and seeing him lie there totally at my mercy was a very strange feeling.

Eventually I decided I had taken him to the top of the scale for long enough, the teasing had worked, and he had reached the point of no return. I glanced over at the clock, he had booked an hour and I had managed to keep him going for the whole time. I released his mouth first, and then undid the rest of the restraints. He thanked me, saying he had enjoyed it very much. In a funny sort of way so had I. He asked if I would consider doing it for him again. I said of course and he left with his two bags either side. I watched him from the window, thinking to myself what a strange request, but then I thought he was happy and it takes all sorts to make a world.

Not long after that scenario, I had a man ring me asking if I would be willing to spank him. This was a new one again, I thought. After my ordeal fending off the bondage man I wondered if I should just say yes, rather than say no, as I hadn't even tried it. After all, I had survived the other strange request, why shouldn't I say yes to this one?

I again explained on the phone about the wheelchair and it didn't seem to bother him in the slightest. We arranged for him to come around the following afternoon. I felt a little anxious, as I certainly didn't want to cause pain to someone, and wasn't sure how far he wanted me to go. He arrived exactly on time, again with a bag. He was a stocky little man, mid fifties, grey hair and chunky arms and legs. He spoke firmly, telling me what I had to do. As he opened the bag, he explained he had brought with him one of his wife's slippers. He said he usually went to another lady who had recently given it up, and that if he liked me he would be coming to see me regularly. He explained he had a high profile job, and was in charge of lots of people. I didn't ask what he did, as I just listened, wondering if this was why he did this kind of thing. Perhaps it was the opposite of the position he held at work.

He instructed me to slap him as hard as I could anywhere between the tops of his buttocks to just above the knees. He told me to slap him as hard as possible with his wife's slipper and order him to do things. "Tell me to get on my knees or whatever you want," he said.

"I will do," I replied.

"Just one more thing," he said. "You must not stop hitting me, no matter what I say, and even if I tell you to stop, you must keep on hitting me until I have been punished. Only then will I shoot my spunk. Do you understand?" he said, looking at me all excited.

"Yes, I understand, if that's what you want I'm prepared to do it."

Only one thing concerned me now and that was the strength in my arms. I am very strong from pushing the wheelchair and I can beat most blokes in an arm wrestle. Therefore I was worried that I might hurt him, and I wasn't sure if he realised this. I had had a rather frustrating day so was rather looking forward to being able to take it out on a willing person. Anyway I ordered him to strip completely naked for me. Then I gave one order after another, telling him sternly, "Get on your knees," and I told him to do as he was told at all times. I said, "Brush the pile on the carpet to the left," then I said, "Brush it to the right," as he was bent over on all fours. Then I would suddenly whack him as hard as I could with the slipper. I whacked his buttocks really hard, over and over, whack, whack, whack, as hard as I could. His cheeks were getting red and his face looked like he was in agony. I then ordered him to stand up in front of me. This time I gently ran my hand between his legs, just lightly touching him, and then suddenly when he wasn't expecting it – whack, I belted his thigh as hard as I could with the slipper over and over. He started pleading with me to stop and I said, "No, you are going to take this punishment." He tried to bend away in an effort to get away from me, so I chased him around the room, whacking even harder than before. When I felt he couldn't take any more, I ordered him to wank off in front of me. It worked; he loved it. I had enjoyed it too, very little work, I figured, for the money, and I had a lot of satisfaction from being so bossy and domineering. He left as another satisfied customer, to return again as a regular.

At times I felt as if I could easily go down the road of domination. I found it easy after the experiences before. Each time it became easier and easier for me. I had wondered if it was to do with the acting I had done previously, giving me the ability to switch from my natural character to someone that I was asked to be. Since my nature is naturally quite bossy, this role was becoming easy to play.

Yet again I was contacted by a so-called slave. This one was even more extreme, and he came with a complete list of instructions. This man was happily married, living a normal life at home, and yet with me he wanted to be the complete opposite. He wanted me to treat him as a complete sissy. He would like to turn up in ladies' knickers under his normal everyday work clothes of a smart suit and tie. After removing the normal clothes he would like to stand in front of me in frilly knickers and knee high white school socks. His request was to respect, worship and obey me at all times as his mistress. He wanted to learn how to humiliate himself in front of me. I had to train him to be a pathetic slut tart.

He had drawn up a list of confessions he must learn and repeat in front of me:

◦ Learn and repeat at any time a 50-word self-scorn description of what a pathetic slut he was;

◦ Learn a stupid little slut song and dance with posing and exposing;

◦ Learn to catwalk like a model;

◦ Learn to talk in a little girl's voice;

◦ Learn to give a running commentary on what he was doing, what he was feeling, and how pathetic he was.

The list was endless and getting more extreme, even saying I had to make him cry in a little girl's voice as I made him parade around the room for me dressed in whatever I required. I had to make him play with his bottom, and then slap his balls as hard as he could take it. Next I had to make him dance for me like a real tart, parading up and down wiggling his hips and arse, as if he was pole dancing without the pole. I had to call out the numbers at random and he would act out that particular request. He would say a prayer of worship to me that he had learnt on arrival. He wasn't sure at what point or how many times I would make him say this, so he had to be prepared and memorise it ready for me. If he let me down in any way, mistress would have to punish him, by making him do disgusting things like sticking his finger up his bottom, and then lick it off, after pretending it was a cock, and sucking it for me. Mistress had to take photographs and could even threaten, that her friends would walk in and watch him acting like a sissy slut too.

The scenarios were endless and it seemed as if there were no boundaries. He loved every second of it. I would ask myself how this normal-looking family man could be into so much obedience as a slave? Over and over I have asked myself how men get into wanting this treatment. I was paid the money and did as instructed, forgetting what is normal and giving the client what he wanted.

Chapter 21
All Kinds

After a year or so of massaging I had got used to seeing all sorts of men. The oldest client was eighty-eight and barely able to make it in the front door, let alone onto the massage table. The youngest was twenty-seven. I have never felt comfortable about seeing young men, as my children are in their twenties and I don't like to think of young men in that way. So by choice I have rejected the younger client.

The first visit was always the hardest for them and for me. As I have said before, it was like being on blind date, not knowing who was going to walk through the door. The voice on the phone very rarely matched the man that walked in. Whilst I waited for them, I would have a mental picture of what I thought they would look like, and I am sure they did the same about me. Very often I would be totally shocked. I would picture, say, a man who had been a little shy on the phone, to be little, and when they walked in they would be completely the opposite. Standing at 6 feet 5 inches and being so large they would struggle to get onto the massage table. My biggest fear would be that they would break the table.

When it came to the point of asking them to turn over, I would grit my teeth and wait for the crunch with bated breath. On one occasion not long after I had ordered a nice new, wider massage table, I had a man turn up who wasn't big or fat, but just got very excited and wriggled around all over the table. Unfortunately this did crack the table and I couldn't believe it. "Oh no," I thought, "my brand new bed, ruined." After that I was always very worried as it wasn't like you could say to someone on the phone, "By the way, are you fat, because if you are I don't want to see you." That would have been rude and discriminating. After all, who was I to judge, as I couldn't even walk.

Only twice did someone book an appointment and leave when they found out I was in a wheelchair. I didn't blame them. I was surprised it didn't happen more often. At least most men gave me a chance, and continued on to be regulars.

Another thing I found was that there are so many different shapes and sizes. I don't just mean in bodies but penises also. Some bend to the left, some to the right, some upright, big, small, medium, I was getting used to all kinds. Some of my clients had been brave to visit me as I have had a few with such tiny penises, but I never flinched or showed any sign of surprise.

One instance that sticks in my mind was a man in his thirties. I though he was the most handsome man I had ever seen, as he removed his clothes and placed them in the chair. I was thinking what a beautiful body he had, great muscles, six pack chest and gorgeous face. He seemed to have it all and I couldn't quite understand why he should need to come and pay for a massage service, when the girls must be fighting over him. I was so shocked when it came to the hand relief part of the massage. He had such a tiny penis that my heart went out to him. I didn't react, but after he left I kept thinking to myself, "How does he get on when he picks up a girl in a nightclub?" I imagined him taking them home and then them finding out what a tiny penis he had, and being thoroughly disappointed. I think it must be worse for a good-looking man to have to deal with that.

The other thing to consider was the cleanliness of the clients. Were the men going to come to you nice and clean, or had they been sweating and not bathed for a day or so? Generally it was OK, but I did have a really bad client one day. He had been trying me for weeks, but we could not get the timing right. Eventually we arranged a time convenient for both of us. It was a Saturday afternoon in the summer. He walked in and I nearly died. The smell immediately hit me like a brick wall, it was stale sweat. He had long hair, dirty clothes on, and hadn't washed for what seemed weeks. I was trapped as he stripped and came towards me to get onto the massage table. I started to panic a little as I wasn't sure if I was going to retch and vomit. I held my breath for as long as I could, but it was impossible so I just took shallow small breaths when I had to. I tried to talk and be nice, but this was making it worse. For the first time ever I had to leave the room during the massage and go and get a drink of water. I was almost praying it could be over sooner than the one hour period he had booked. Now it got to the crucial moment, when I had to get him to turn over. I really didn't want this bit to come, as I knew it meant touching his penis. The rest of him was bad enough and I really wasn't sure how I was going to deal with that.

Suddenly my mobile rang. I don't usually answer it when I am with a client, but on this occasion I did. It was a call to say my dad had been taken ill, and I had to get to the hospital quick. This was terrible news but in some ways it was such a relief as I told the man that I was sorry but he had to go as I had an emergency. I refunded him the money, he got dressed and left in a hurry with me apologising. Phew, I had been given a lucky escape on that occasion. It was such a bad experience that it made me wonder how the women offering a full personal service would have dealt with that sort of client. Luckily that was my worst hygiene experience, and I was saved.

Chapter 22
Don't Mess with a Masseuse

Dealing with money was always a tricky subject, even when someone was paying you for a service you had provided. I soon learnt that there were some men that thought they could have something for nothing. One particular afternoon a person I thought to be a gentleman turned up for a massage. On arrival he was very smartly dressed in a suit and tie. He was well spoken and seemed a grateful client. Throughout the massage he was considerate and never tried to push past the boundaries of expecting anything other than a massage with relief. On leaving he paid me and left, as I used to take the payment after the massage rather than before. Firstly because I trusted them to pay, and secondly because I felt it would be better for them to pay me after, just in case they had not been happy with my service for any reason. However I soon learnt the hard way that this was not a good idea.

That evening the telephone rang. It was him thanking me for a wonderful massage and he was full of compliments. He continued to tell me how good it made him feel and that he hadn't felt like that in a long time. This was very encouraging, although not unusual to have them call me up later to thank me. I returned the compliment, telling him it was a pleasure to meet him. He had rung me from a private withheld number and again at the time I used to accept these calls. However this was also something I soon learnt to change.

A few weeks later, one evening at around 7 o'clock the phone rang from a private number. I answered it and it was him, and he sounded in a bit of a state. I had had a hard day, and was exhausted from working. I had not eaten and had just a few minutes earlier ordered a Chinese takeaway. He was begging me for an appointment, telling me he had had such a bad day, that his father had been taken into hospital and that he was in desperate need of a soothing massage and someone to talk to. I explained that I didn't really have any appointments left and that I had ordered my Chinese and was waiting for it to be delivered any second. However he wasn't accepting no for an answer, begging me and making me feel guilty. In the end I suggested I could put the Chinese meal in the oven whilst I did his massage, and with that suggestion he came round within five minutes of hanging up the phone.

So with the meal in the oven I let my heart rule my head and executed the massage for him. The time was extended a little as he was telling me all about his father being so ill and in the hospital etc. I listened sympathetically, gave him kind words of comfort and generally made him feel welcome. Although I had sacrificed my meal by another hour and a half, I looked after him how I felt I would have wanted to be treated under those conditions.

It was time for him to leave and he got dressed again in his smart clothes. He then tapped his pocket and said, "Oh dear, I appear to have left my wallet at the hospital." At the time I was concerned not so much for my money, but by the fact that if his wallet was left in the hospital, it might have gone missing by now. I advised him to go straight back and see if it had been found. He seemed rather laid back about this suggestion and said, "Oh, don't worry, I'll get it tomorrow."

"Tomorrow?" I said. "That's not a good idea. I think you should go straight back to A & E, because if they move your dad to a ward you may never find it."

Again he didn't seem to want to even try. I offered to let him ring them from my phone to see if it had been handed in. However he just wanted to leave and not take any action to find it that evening. "I'll pay you tomorrow," he said as he put his coat on.

"Just one thing," I replied. "Can I have your mobile number as it's been coming up as withheld."

"Yes," he replied and started giving me the first few digits and then stopped. He said, "I tell you what, I will give you a ring in a second from the car, and then the number will come up on your phone." I had caller display so I could see who was calling before I answered.

"OK," I replied, and let him go. "Good luck with finding your wallet," I said as he went out, "and don't forget to call me from the car." I waved him off as he walked out of the door.

A few minutes later the phone rang and the number was withheld. I answered it and it was him. "Your number hasn't come up again," I said.

He replied, "Oh, never mind, I'll pop the money in tomorrow," and he hung up without me being able to say another word.

I went to the oven to find my Chinese takeaway was ruined. Here I was, still hungry. I had just worked for another hour and a half and not a penny better off. Still, I thought I would be paid for that tomorrow.

Tomorrow came and went without as much as a phone call from him, let alone the money he owed me. That evening I became angry, as I realised that I had been taken advantage of. I would rather give someone something than have them take it like that. I felt so cross that I had even sacrificed not just my time for him but also my food. In fact I had also wasted the money I had used to pay for the food, and now here he was taking the piss. I found the piece of paper I had used to start writing down his phone number, and there were three digits missing from the end. My only hope was that I could work out the right combination. I was so determined to find these last digits. After a few hours and a few calls to wrong numbers I had worked it out. I narrowed it down to about six numbers. Some I ruled out straight away, for instance if it had a woman's voice mail or even a man's voice that I did not recognise. I had six left to try but thought I would wait until the morning. I was on a mission and by now it wasn't even the money, it was the principle.

The next day at about 10 am, I tried the last few, when bingo,

I found him. I recognised his voice straight away, but he didn't recognise mine. "Hello, how are you?" I asked.

With that he replied as if he thought I was someone he knew: "I'm fine, thanks."

"What are you doing today?" I asked.

"Nothing," he replied. "Do you want to come over?"

"Oh yes," I replied and then he went on to say, "Your voice sounds a bit different today, are you OK?" I thought shit, he has sussed it out, but luckily he hadn't as he went on to say, "I thought you had to work today?"

I replied, "Yes I did, but I am off with a bad throat." He asked me what time could I come over and shall we go out.

Then I asked, "How's your dad?"

"Oh, he's fine," he replied. "He had the doctor out the other day but he's not too bad at all."

With that I couldn't keep up the pretend voice any longer. I said, "Really, so he's not in hospital then?"

"Who is this?" he replied. With that I put the phone down.

A few seconds later I rang back and started asking more questions. He kept asking me who I was and I started laughing and saying, "You really don't know, do you?"

"No," he said. "Who the hell is it?"

With that I said plainly, "You owe me some money from the other night, don't you?"

He replied in a state of shock, "How did you get my number?"

"Never mind that," I replied. "Not only do I know your phone number, but I have also traced where you live. So if you don't bring me my money before 12 pm today, someone will be calling at your house to collect it."

He stammered, "OK, I'll bring it round, I promise."

I said, "OK, but just one more thing, don't post it through the letter box. I want you to knock on the door and give it to me in person." He agreed and I put the phone down.

At 11.50 the next day he pulled up outside my house. He walked up to the door and tried to lift up the letter box to post it. I had the camera on and was recording so I could see him. With that I quickly opened the door. He looked at me, totally shocked, tried apologising and telling me more sob stories about how he had had to go and put flowers on his sister's grave. This time I had no sympathy for his tales of woe. I said, "Cut the crap, I heard enough of it the night before last. Just give me the money you owe me and don't bother ringing me again." With that he left.

After that experience I had to ask myself, "Do I trust people too damn much, that someone could take my kindness and abuse it?" However it did teach me to always take payment first and not to accept a booking from a withheld number, as you just cannot rely on trust in this type of work.

Chapter 23
Meeting Mike

It was on Friday the 21st of May 2004, just two days after the report had gone on the website and just one day after my birthday. I received a call from a man called Mike. He sounded quite excitable on the phone, he talked fast and asked if he could come along. I replied yes of course and within about twenty minutes there was a knock at the door.

He came in rather like a hurricane, full of excitement and enthusiasm and tearing his clothes off as fast as he could. I don't think I had ever seen anyone as keen. I remember thinking he was rather a scruffy looking man, who didn't seem to care too much about his appearance, or his clothes. He had dark hair which was very untidy and all over the place. Not shaved for a day or so and just didn't seem bothered. Even though he knew he was going to visit a lady, it didn't seem important to him what he looked like. Me being me, I tried not to judge, as I thought if he was kind enough to call and pay me for a massage then I should be grateful. After all, when the half hour was up he would be gone and why should it matter to me what the hell anyone looks like?

He climbed onto the massage couch and asked if I could leave the big light on. This was something which I had never been asked to do before. Anyway I respected his wishes and it became very clear from the beginning that he didn't want any sort of massage. He asked me if I could put a bra on and just lean over him playing with his nipples. OK, I thought, if that's what you want I shall oblige. I went into the bedroom to put on a bra for him, a red one. I went back to the massage couch and did exactly as he asked.

I started off by gently rubbing his nipples and showing him my cleavage. He was getting more excited by the second. He commented on my eyes, telling me how beautiful they were. I looked at his smiling face and encouraged him too with naughty words, getting him more excited by the second. He asked me to kiss him and I said just a peck, as I didn't like kissing people, it wasn't part of my service. He asked me to tease him by showing him my tongue, and I did this for him. I found this really fun, as he was just so easy to please. After the half hour he had shot his load and he seemed grateful. As he was getting dressed he was briefly telling me he lived with someone, but wasn't happy, as they hadn't had sex for years. I listened as I did with all my clients, saying yes and no in the right places and showing sympathy where needed. Then he left in pretty much the same hurry as he had entered.

The next time I heard from Mike was just one week and a day later, on Saturday the 29th of May. Pretty much the same procedure as the time before, only this time he asked me if I could have my bra on for him when he arrived. I agreed and was waiting ready as he walked in. Again he came in like a hurricane, ripping off his clothes and leaping onto the massage couch. I remembered what he liked, so I left the big light on and teased him again with my tongue. I looked deep into his eyes as I encouraged him with naughty talk, and told him the things he wanted to hear. He loved cleavage and underwear and wanted me to tease his nipples. Again he shot his load as before and seemed so grateful. Again as he was getting dressed we talked a little more. He seemed such a desperate man, full of sorrow about his relationship. He said he liked me and said I was very good at my job, even though I didn't do full sex. He said I was better than most of the girls he had visited before. He asked if he could pay me £10 extra and call me up some time for a dirty phone chat. I accepted but I did ask him how we would go about it, as it wasn't easy to plan it his end or mine, as I might be working when he needed me. He understood this and said he would take the risk.

He had obviously done this sort of thing before, and many years ago for a few months I had done some phone work for a man in Bradford, called Call Backs. Basically you would pretend to be whatever they requested. The man in Bradford would tell you the age and colour that you must pretend to be. Everything was all picked by this man, all I had to do was pretend to be that woman, so I was kind of used to talking dirty if I needed to.

A few days later, his number was calling my phone. I was alone with no clients so I answered him. It was the dirty phone chat he wanted. I obliged by doing the same trick for him. After we had talked for just a few minutes he was calling me by my name. He asked if I owned a white lacy bra for his next visit. I didn't but I did promise I would buy one for him. The next day I kept my promise and went to the shops, hunting for the best bra I could find. Don't ask me why I was doing this for a client. I had never done this before, well not that I had been asked to. But for some reason with Mike I felt I wanted to help him. I was in Beales and I had just paid for the bra when my phone rang and it was Mike. Oh no, I thought, I couldn't do a phone chat now. I answered it anyway to say sorry I am out. He was in a bit of a state. "What's the matter?" I asked. He went on to explain that after our phone chat the day before, his daughter had been in the house and heard him. She thought he was having an affair. "Oh no," I said, "how awful." He said she heard him say my name and everything. I felt terrible for him and didn't know what to do to help. I said just tell her the truth; tell her how it was, nothing more than a couple of dirty phone chats. He agreed, and later he explained to her the situation between himself and her mother. She did seem to understand, and the matter was dropped.

Mike continued to come round and see me, having the usual service, sometimes paying me a little extra for the phone chat. We started to talk more after each visit and I would allow him to stay well over his time as I felt so sorry for him. He seemed so desperately sad about his relationship. He wasn't married to her but they had a son between them. It seemed that since his son was born, sex was off the menu, leaving him to satisfy himself. We talked about his children, he was so proud of them both; even though his daughter wasn't his child he loved her just the same as his son. His daughter liked singing, so Mike and I had a major talking point. I had a tape in my stereo unit which I had recorded a few years ago. I played it to him and he sat there crying, saying how wonderful my voice was. He said you have it all, the beautiful big blue eyes that just capture everyone and the fantastic personality. He said, "You should do more with your singing, the public would love you."

I said, "I would have liked to, but by now my job would probably be to my detriment."

Sometimes we would talk for an hour after the booking time was up. I tried so hard to help him in his relationship back home. I suggested he just sit her down and talk to her, telling her everything. I told him to tell her how he felt and that he had needs. He agreed, saying he would try. I wished him good luck as he left.

I think from that moment on I felt different towards Mike. My heart went out to him. He had it all at home; he had a swimming pool, jacuzzi, and four-bedroom house. But to look at him he seemed to have nothing at all. He seemed sad, and in desperate need of someone to love and care for him.

The next time he came to me he said the talk had not worked at all. He said she even said to him to go and find someone else to make him happy. I was really surprised, but not knowing both sides of the story it is always so hard to judge and I didn't know her. However I was beginning to know Mike. I kept making suggestions to try and help, but nothing worked. I began to see why he didn't make an effort with his appearance, as he didn't have a lot of self-esteem. He was an electronic design engineer, good at his job, and very positive where work was concerned.

I didn't see Mike for a few weeks. I can't remember why, either I was busy when he rang or I was having a day off. When I did see him again we did the usual things he liked. We talked after, only this time he was begging me to sleep with him, pleading and saying I will pay you more. I kept saying no, but a little part of me felt so cruel for saying no when I knew he was rejected at home. I knew he visited other prostitutes, but he said they were cold and not caring. He said they did the business, but were not there for him like I was. They just took the money and didn't care a damn. This played on my mind, although it shouldn't have since after all he was just a client. But for some reason I did care about him. My husband Colin was aware of Mike and his situation at home. I think he felt for him too being rejected. I had told Colin about my intentions for Mike, and how I wanted to be there for him and help him. Colin did not ever object to my relationship with Mike. Mike and I exchanged email addresses (actually I set up a special one that only he knew about). He would write to me nearly every day, telling me all about his past and how he had a broken marriage of eighteen years. He would write about his past sex life or lack of it. He just kept writing and pouring out everything from his heart into his emails to me.

I did care, but always tried to keep a bit of me back. Mike was thirteen years older than me, not that this made any difference, as he didn't look or act it.

Chapter 24
Sleeping with Mike

I continued to see Mike for about a year on and off. However one day marked a big turning point in my life. He had rung as usual and came in again like a hurricane, full of excitement. Only this time I said to him, "Do you remember the offer you made me last time, Mike? Would you still like to have full sex with me?"

He nearly fainted. I was about to break my golden rule after all these months. Was I mad? Would I live with myself for going that one step further? I didn't have a clue. Was I doing it to help him? I felt sorry for him going to different girls, and feeling awful afterwards. All these things were running through my head, and I was feeling scared. Although I knew him, I was very self-conscious of my body, and especially being paid. It wasn't like being on a date when you sleep with a bloke and then never see them again if neither of you like each other. This was a business arrangement even if we were friends. It wasn't an affair that would be wrong from both our sides with me married and him living with someone.

After I said I would sleep with him, he shot out the door, running over to the cash point machine to draw out some more money. I have never seen a man as keen in my entire life as he was that day. I was waiting for him in the bedroom. He was ripping off his trousers in such a hurry his credit and bank cards fell out of his pocket onto the floor. I said, "Hey, steady on, you are losing your cards." He didn't even seem to care, as there was only one thought on his mind.

As he climbed on top of me, asking me to rub his nipples, I placed the condom onto his hard cock and glided it into me.

"Tell me you love me," he begged me. I couldn't and I didn't.

"Please," he begged me, "say you love me."

"Oh my god," I thought, "this is awful, how can I tell a man fucking me for money that I love him when I don't?" At that point I knew I had to lie, after all he was paying me. So I said the difficult words and thought I would explain later. Now was not the time to talk sensibly. As I said the words he climaxed and then cuddled me saying, "Thank you so much." He seemed truly grateful. I explained it was hard for me to say I loved him, but I hoped it helped him to come.

I said, "I don't like to say those words unless I mean them." He did understand and explained it had been so long since someone had said that to him. He just felt it would be nice to hear me say them as he knew I did care a lot and we had built up a good friendship.

I had some other massage bookings so after we talked for a while Mike had to go, I had to remind him to pick up his cards off my bedroom floor, and we still laugh about that to this day.

He wanted to carry on seeing me like this on a regular basis. Part of me wished I had not done it, as now I felt I had crossed the line. I had moments of dread and very bad thoughts about how low I had sunk. What would people think of me, especially my family? But it was too late. I had done it and there was no going back. He had been a few more times, and also put a report on the site like Shaun had, telling people how good I was, but not mentioning the full personal as I didn't want that on there.

One Saturday Mike rang me to see how I was, and I was in a bit of a state as I was having problems with a new electric wheelchair I had bought with a bank loan. After having the chair three weeks I found I couldn't get on with it at all. It was a totally different style and type to the one I had had before and I now hated it. I rang the shop up and asked if could I swap it for one like I had had before, and they said yes, no problem. However the only thing was, there was a £1,000 difference in the price. I was stuck, as the money from the loan was gone and I didn't have enough to get the other chair. At that point I didn't have a clue what to do. Mike was very sympathetic on the phone and without a word of hesitation offered – and I repeat *offered* – to lend me the £1,000 to put towards the chair I wanted. I couldn't believe it. Within half an hour he was at my door holding the money, together with a huge Easter egg. I have never seen such kindness in a man who had not hesitated in offering his help.

We had agreed it would be a loan and he would now not pay to see me until the money had been used up in his visits. The first visit was very soon, within a few days. It went OK, the same as before only on this occasion he didn't seem to respect the time factor. After the hour was up I kindly mentioned I had another booking and must not be much longer. He complained, saying, "I wish I'd known that in the beginning." I apologised, but stated I had also to do other work. In the back of my mind I thought, "It is all well and good lending me the £1,000, but if I am unable to fit the rest of my regulars into a morning, it will be hard trying to meet my other commitments." After an hour and a half I finally persuaded him to go. I could see he didn't like it, and at the time it made me quite mad.

That day I thought more and more about it, and ended up writing him an email explaining that I was grateful for what he had done for me. However, unless we stuck to the agreed time of an hour, I could not accept this arrangement. The thought of owing him all that money did in fact make me panic, knowing I was now committed to sleeping with him to pay it back. The thought really did scare me and I regretted making the agreement. Also I could see he was going to be very demanding of my time.

After the email he rang me and we had a rather heated discussion, with him telling me that when he had visited one or two other girls before, they would not worry about the time. I kept explaining that if it was going to work with us, we would both have to realise it would be for only an hour, and that way we would both know from the outset where we were. I could then plan the rest of my day, and after each visit cross off the agreed amount owing. He accepted reluctantly. On several occasions he would ring to come and see me, and I would state a time, but he would ask if he could come around earlier and just watch me getting ready. I was horrified at this and said, "No, please Mike, don't turn up any earlier than the agreed time." I didn't want him here watching me get ready.

This was just the start of Mike and me falling out. He was on the other hand very generous, and we had continued to write to each other on a daily basis. He tried to help me as a friend whenever possible, sometimes showering me with gifts. He bought me a printer, a camera, huge bars of chocolates and cards containing the most meaningful words. I couldn't believe how he had found these most precious meaningful words in a card. When it came to my Birthday he said he wanted to give me something personal. He had gone to the jeweller's and found a locket in the shape of a heart and had arranged for my name to be engraved down one side.

It was beautiful and we were starting to get closer. I remember one night, all his family had gone away for the weekend, leaving him at home alone. It was nice as I could call him freely and we could talk when ever we wanted. We started talking on the phone one Sunday night at about ten o'clock in the evening, and we were still talking at four the next morning. We talked about everything from my childhood to the present day, and likewise he confided in me about his personal feelings. He normally went to sleep at ten every night, but on this occasion he just wanted to keep on talking. He had taken the phone into the bedroom and was lying there talking, and telling me how much he liked me.

I wasn't sure at this point if I had made a mistake. I didn't usually let down my barriers to people very easily, even though he had been a wonderful friend. He was always there on the end of an email or text. Now I felt he was starting to know more about me and my life than I had really wanted him to. After all I had to remember he was still a paying client. Not only that, but Mike had a unique knack of saying or doing things to upset me. One of the biggest fall-outs we had was over the particular website he had put a report on about me. He said he would write another one to try and help, particularly as he felt it was all true. After he posted this report, the website got very upset as he was not supposed to have posted another one within such a short time period. Therefore they suspended his profile and in the process also took off both his new and his original reports about me. This now meant it looked bad on my side at now having lost instead of gaining a rating. I was very upset with him. So upset that I asked him if he knew of any other websites where I could advertise myself. He suggested a couple and apologised for messing up my other site. I finished the call from him and then looked up the sites he had suggested. A few days later he managed to get back the original report after sending a grovelling email to the site organiser.

Chapter 25
Me as an Escort

I was not very computer literate but did my best to fumble around. There were the sites that Mike had mentioned. I studied very hard on what they were all about and came to the conclusion that they were all prostitute's sites, advertising only one thing. No in-between or massaging, just full-blown sex. Next I found myself registering, not having a clue if I was doing it right or even if I should. The form-filling was done and the next thing I remember was that I was now a member offering services. Quite what yet I hadn't decided. It was asking me to write up my profile, add pictures, and say what I was offering. Within a few hours I had gone from never hearing about this site to being a fully fledged member, although the bonus was it was free to join.

I studied a lot of the girls already advertising on there and saw how they came across. Some were so gorgeous I wished I could have been like them. Then at the other extreme there were just ordinary women, older and younger, who weren't supermodels, just women offering sex. Prostitutes had always fascinated me. I remember if I had ever been driven past an area where girls were working I would glance over and look. I was not sure what I was expecting to see, but the whole idea did interest me. The other part of me looked at these women and thought, "Well, I suppose I am already a prostitute, as I've been sleeping with Mike now for months, and taking money for it."

It was getting late now and the evening had flown by, although I was still being driven to carry on with my profile that

I had started. I had decided to go for it, and before I knew it I was ticking certain boxes saying what services I was offering, the whole works. The other problem was that I didn't want to deceive people that looked at my profile, so I called myself "Something different". Then I went on to write about being in a wheelchair. I felt nervous, but a little part of me felt excited too. I was also cross at Mike for messing up the other site, as I needed the money and heavily relied on the reports to give me business. Now I was going down a different road. One I didn't want to tell anybody about, not even Mike.

The next day I woke up early, logged into my profile and couldn't believe my eyes. I had hundreds of emails from men asking to see me. Some saying they didn't mind me being in a wheelchair, and some even saying they had always had a fantasy about fucking someone in that situation. In fact they would apologise for having such thoughts, all of which I found funny, and didn't take too seriously.

Before I knew it I had my first real booking, a man who lived thirty miles away. I got myself all ready, and not having a clue really if I looked OK for him. Next I could see him walking up the path. I took a big breath and thought, "Oh well, here goes." My heart was in my mouth in case he didn't like me.

I greeted him nervously, shaking his hand and pretending I knew what I was doing. "Would you like to start with a massage?" I offered as he stripped off in front of me. He didn't seem at all nervous as he revealed a huge hard cock to me. I did the usual things I had been used to doing, gently massaging and teasing, only this time I knew I was being paid for everything. I wasn't sure about how to go about leaving the massage table and entering the bedroom and getting on the bed.

Soon the decision was taken out of my hands, as after a few moment of playing with his enormous hard cock, he started to rub his hand over my open cleavage. I was wearing a black Basque, and stockings and suspenders under my skirt. He asked if I was able to get up onto the massage table. I replied, "Yes, if that is what you would like." He nodded and I lifted myself from my chair and onto the massage table, grabbing the condom from the side of my bag as I went. As I got onto the table he stood in front of me, admiring me like I was a doll or something, stroking my face, and telling me what lovely eyes I had. He then proceeded to pull my tits out of my Basque and cup them between his hands, caressing them, and squeezing my nipples until he could see how much I was enjoying it. He gently lowered me onto my back, lifting my skirt up and with my legs either side of him. He was looking down at my pussy which was now very wet. He touched me and it felt so good. I felt so naughty, as if I should not have been doing this terrible thing and yet here I was enjoying the naughtiness of it. What a fantasy, I thought, a complete stranger has come here, given me money, and is now giving me a real good time.

His mouth went down onto my breasts, as I felt his fingers enter me. He lowered his hot breath onto my now very open and exposed cunt, and started licking me intensely. I could feel I was going to come. "I want to fuck you now," he whispered in my ear. That was it, I couldn't hold it back any more. It was too many fantasies in one go, the naughtiness of the situation, and a complete stranger whispering in my ear. Suddenly I gushed all over his face and down my legs. After drinking up all my juices he could take from me, he held his big hard cock ready for me to place the condom on, and then inserted it up inside me. Groaning and jerking, fucking me harder and harder on the massage table, his back arched and he let out an almighty noise.

I was now officially a hooker.

Chapter 26
Falling out with Mike

A few days later, I had had a booking placed for a certain time and date, quite unusually, as most of the bookings came direct from phone calls rather than through the booking system. Anyway I made a note of the number, which appeared to have a lot of zeros in it.

The next day I had a call from a very cross Mike. I had not actually spoken to him for about three weeks, with one thing and another. My close friend Nigel had at the time been in hospital dying from cancer, and so when I wasn't working I was sitting with him trying to comfort him. I remember looking at him just before he finally died, thinking, "Oh dear, I hope you never get to hear what I have been doing." I think it would have broken his heart, as he had always cared for me. Unfortunately I wasn't attracted to him, so it would have really hurt him to think I was willing to sleep with strangers for money. However my worry was over regarding him finding out about my recent events, as sadly he passed away within four days.

Mike was livid with me, asking, "Why didn't you tell me that you had gone onto the site that I told you about?"

I went silent, and then replied, "How did you find out?"

"I saw you on there," he said. He went on to explain how hurt he was that I had done that to him. He said, "I thought I was the only one who paid you for sex."

"You were," I explained, but he wasn't happy at all.

He said, "I've put a bloody booking in." Everything now fell into place. It was him who placed the phoney phone number with all the zeros in it, it didn't actually exist.

We had some cross words, with me telling him it was really not anything to do with him what I did. I also told him that it was entirely his fault in the first place. After all it was him who encouraged me to do it in the first place, and it was also him who messed up my report on the original site. He seemed very upset and jealous. I could not accept this attitude from a client/friend or anyone else who tried to make a judgement on my life. I had thought long and bloody hard about it. I didn't find it easy and certainly didn't want to be told by a client who was in a relationship already that I was not to do this with anyone else for money.

The next time I saw Mike was the 1st of April and he seemed to have accepted the fact that I was on the site as a prostitute. In fact that day he arrived with a box of chocolates and gave me the money, despite me still owing him from the loan. We talked about recent events, and what I had been up to with other men. This seemed to excite Mike rather than make him mad. Whilst he was here, he wanted me to talk about what I had had done and ended up getting more and more turned on. He seemed to be accepting the situation and that day we had some fantastic sex.

We both fulfiled our secret fantasies. Mike had always fantasised about naughty girls, especially prostitutes, throughout his life. In turn I had always liked the idea of fucking a stranger. Now our fantasies were merging into one. The following Sunday I knew Mike's family were away, and I woke up feeling extremely horny. A few minutes later the phone rang and it was him. I asked if he would like to come round for the morning with no time limit and no charge. He jumped at it and was here in my bed within a few minutes of my offer. We spent the whole morning having fun and then lying there talking. For the first time ever, I wasn't in a hurry for him to go. He did leave at about lunch time however, as I had some friends turning up in the afternoon.

We carried on emailing, and he carried on helping me. In fact he bought me a digital camera so I could take some pictures for my website. He also purchased a printer/scanner as he wanted me to send over some photos via email to him whenever I could. Mike became Mr Reliable. If he said he was going to do something he always did it, and at that point he had never let me down. We grew closer and I stopped keeping an account of how many times we slept together. He often called in on the way home from work, at weekends, and whenever he could escape from home without too much suspicion.

A few weeks later I had a hospital appointment as I had been suffering with a kidney problem for many years. Mike was waiting for an email to say I was OK, but when I got home I felt so ill I didn't turn on the computer, which worried him and caused him to ring round the hospitals to see if I was still there. Of course I wasn't, I was tucked up at home in bed. The next day Mike and I fell out again, which I could fully understand as I should have told him. The biggest problem Mike and I had at this point was his mouth and lack of thinking before he spoke. The other problem was that he was getting possessive.

One of the biggest things that hurt me at this point was his habit of making comments without thinking. There was one comment that I have never and will never forget. It was a personal comment about my body and I immediately got upset, but tried to hide it when he was still with me. Later I emailed him, telling him I didn't ever want to sleep with him again as I didn't feel good enough and that he should go and find himself another prostitute. He rang me from outside his work in a terrible state, crying and telling me he was sorry. I agreed to still be friends after a two-hour conversation, although I still told him he was to go and find another woman to sleep with.

I stuck to this for a while. One Saturday not long after, he arranged to see a lady from the paper. I was so glad, and told him he could call in on the way home to see me as a friend if he wished. When he arrived he looked sad, and I asked him how it went. He replied, "It's no good, I don't want her, I want you." Seeing the sadness in his eyes I truly believed him, and again felt sorry for him. I did forgive him after that and we continued as before. Only this time I was seeing more clients than ever.

Chapter 27
Phone Chats & Web Cam

I remember the first time I ever logged on for phone chats using this new site. One, I felt extremely nervous and two, I wasn't sure if anyone would book me. The system was rather tricky to work out; how to accept a booking, take the payment, and have it ready for the caller before it timed out. Before I did this I searched around the site looking at the other girls who were offering services like phone chat and also web cam.

I was so fascinated by this new adventure. I started reading some of the really pretty girls' ratings, as this was something people could put on about you, after you had provided a service for them. It was a way for clients to tell others if they were happy with what you had offered, if you did it well and if they would return. There were three boxes to tick: negative, neutral and positive, and a section to leave a few comments. I was quite envious at that time as I didn't have any ratings as I had not been on there long enough to offer either escort, phone chat, or web cam.

I continued to look through the advertised girls, and I remember looking at one particular girl's profile about one in the morning. I found her really attractive and she had a lot of good ratings. I could see she had also done bookings for web cam and phone chats for ladies as well as men. My heart was racing as I wanted to book her, but wasn't sure how the system worked. Eventually I plucked up the courage and put in a booking, and within minutes she had emailed me back and accepted. The only problem was I wasn't sure how to transfer the credits and the booking timed out before I figured it out. After a few emails from her, and a lot of understanding, I managed to work it out, and she did the web cam show for me. Her words to me were reassuring as she carried on emailing me through MSN for an hour after the booking. She said when you have been doing this for a while it will become easy; her words were comforting and so very true.

I decided the next day to advertise myself for phone chat. Within a few minutes I had a booking come through. Fumbling my way around the computer I accepted the booking and within a few more minutes the phone I had chosen to use for this service began to ring.

Seductively I answered it, saying my name in a sultry voice and asking, "What would you like to talk about?" My imagination suddenly went into autopilot. The voice on the other end of the phone was breathing heavily. He asked what I was wearing, so I said, "A black basque, black stockings, etc." I tried to think of all the things a man would want to hear, and truly believe. It worked, he did believe it. "Tell me more," he said excitedly. I told him I was lying on the bed looking at myself in the mirror, playing with myself, and wishing he was here with me right now. I told him how I would gently remove his trousers and reveal his hard throbbing cock. His excitement grew more and more, as I described how I would suck his cock and look into his face with my big blue eyes, whilst he came in my mouth. Suddenly I heard a huge groan from the end of the phone as he shot his load.

Silence followed for a few seconds from his end, and then he politely said, "Thank you very much, that was good." We talked for just a little while after as I wanted to make sure he was happy with my service. He ended up putting a nice rating on for me.

This may have been my first phone chat session but it certainly wasn't my last. I started to build up a lot of confidence, as a lot of men would come back over and over again. I was learning what kind of fantasies men have in their heads. Some would be so extreme. I had thought before I did this job that I was very open-minded, but this was a real eye-opener. I would log on as available at every opportunity I had, the bookings kept coming and so did the men on the end of the phone. I started to build up my profile to fit around my requests, and therefore made up a list of phone chat scenarios that had been requested, plus ones that might bring in the business from my own imagination. On the list I had been running up a huge list of topics.

A very popular one was to be a secret wank at work. I would have the men book me from their computer in the office, and then run down to the toilet with the phone in their hand ready to ring me. I would be their fantasy right there and then in the toilet, whilst they wanked themselves off.

The list was getting bigger and bigger, I learnt that a lot of men like to fantasise about having sex with either their mother, sister, auntie or any other member of the family. My role was becoming greater and so too my imagination. I would get one booking after another, so on one call I might have had to be some one's sister then the next I would have to switch to being Auntie Molly. I would have to act out some of these situations seriously, as if they were really happening. I believed strongly it was the best way, as the men kept coming back for more. I tried my best to always make them happy and tell them what they wanted to hear.

On a lot of occasions I would be booked for an hour at a time. This role was very taxing on me as I had to keep the scenario going all the time, remembering what I had said and thinking about where the fantasy would go next. One evening I was booked by the same man three times, each consisting of one hour. He ended up talking out his fantasy for a total of three hours. He wanted me to be a total slut, and one of the things he liked was to have me all dressed up in a business suit, smart blouse, short skirt, stockings, the lot. He wanted me to get fucked and shoot spunk all over my nice clean clothes, and then to go out shopping with him, knowing I was covered in his spunk. We would then go on to involve other people as we would go to a night club and pick up other men and ladies. It would all end up in one mass orgy. Great, and I must say, to have done that for real would have been fun too.

My ratings were by now going up into the hundreds, all good and positive comments which I found very encouraging. I gathered I must have been saying the right things or they wouldn't have said such good things about me and returned so often. I was now learning different roles again as I found some men wanted me to treat them really badly. One man booked me, asking me not to be at all nice to him. He said, "I want you to swear and call me horrible names." He wanted me to humiliate him, telling him he was pathetic. I quite liked this as I can be very assertive when I want to be. It did the trick as he booked me every night for ages. It was always just a short booking, but he knew just what he wanted. I had to take this call in the living room as I was worried my neighbours would hear me shouting abuse, and wonder what the hell I was doing.

I would go from call to call, switching roles to suit the booking. At times it was difficult as I would go from being a mistress and disciplining in one call, to being used and abused in the next. Neither of which I minded, but I had to concentrate hard to remember which role I was playing. One really extreme scenario was a caller who had a huge fantasy about dogs. He would do most of the talking, and would like me to look at particular internet sites as he told me what he would like to do with the dog. I didn't find this to be my ideal, but I did try to cater for every scenario without too much judgment.

I had also learnt to put on a number of different voices, something I didn't know I could do until the phone chat work started. I could sound very young to extremely posh, depending on the scenario.

I had another regular who for some reason was very negative towards his wife. He would ask me if I would tell him to do horrible things to her, I obliged by telling him he had to spunk in her milk or make her a nasty drink, consisting of spunk or urine. He loved it, and over and over would return for more nasty suggestions, and would get off on the idea. I never asked if he did it for real as I would rather feel he kept it just as a fantasy, although I cannot understand why anyone would want to be so cruel to their wife.

Another one who seemed to be against his partner wanted her to be downstairs with her friends when he called me. I was then to make him dare to do things like wank at the top of the stairs, in the fear that his wife or her friend might catch him. He would then shoot his load all down the staircase. On one occasion I could hear her calling him, and I wasn't sure what was going to happen. With that the phone went dead and I never knew if he was in big trouble for being caught red-handed wanking on the stairs.

Another caller liked to dress up in sexy ladies' underwear and I had to make him do things whilst he was looking like a sissy. So I instructed him to go over to the window and open the curtains wide and leave the light on. Therefore if anyone was walking past they could glance over and see him and this used to turn him on immensely. He would then have to tell me when somebody had actually walked by and looked at him. All excited he would say to me, "They are looking at me now, what do you want me to do?" I would tell him to lift his skirt up and show them his silky knickers, and I would ask if they were still looking. "Yes they are," he replied in frenzy. "Well," I said, "give them what they want to see, take out your cock, bend over and wank yourself off so they can see you." With that he did and came with an almighty explosion. I am not sure if there were really people walking past looking or if it was as much in his imagination as mine, but he was another very satisfied customer.

I am often a naughty Nanny too who catches naughty men peeping at the ladies in the hockey changing room. This man has to be punished by being made to wear the short skirt, white blouse, and white socks, and being made to wank himself off in front of all the ladies he had been spying on. In turn they laugh at him as I tell him off and spank him really hard. Sometimes if he is really naughty, Nanny will catch him wanking in the wood wearing a dress. This goes down a treat!

Auntie was very popular with one particular man. He would want to be about eighteen and come to stay over at naughty Auntie's house for the summer holidays. There was a twist though as Auntie was not getting enough sex from her husband. In fact she was totally frustrated, so when her nephew came to stay all her sexual desires were fulfiled. He had secretly always fancied her but had never said anything. This particular summer when he came over, Auntie was standing on a chair wearing a short skirt and a tight pair of knickers as she was cleaning the top of the cupboard. He couldn't help but stare up her skirt as he talked to her. She noticed he was looking, and found this very arousing. Lifting her leg up a bit higher onto the unit so he could see even further, she pretended she was unaware of any sexual thoughts between them, and tried to talk normally. The evidence was getting hard to hide on both sides, as she could feel the juices between her legs staining her knickers. He must have noticed, as when she looked down at him his trousers were bulging with hard cock. He was transfixed by her tight wet gusset. Auntie could not contain her feelings any longer, so climbing down off the chair she asked if he liked what he had seen. Shyly he replied, "Sorry Auntie, but I could not help but look up your skirt and see your wet panties."

"That's OK," she replied and then went on to tell him how she and his uncle were not getting on very well at the moment, and that they hadn't had sex in a long time.

She goes on to explain how she is frustrated constantly, and when she caught him looking up her skirt, it turned her on. She then takes hold of his hand and places it between her breasts. He now can't control himself any longer and picks her up and places her over the kitchen table, spreading her legs wide open and looking directly at her wet juicy cunt. He bends down and starts to kiss her thighs, telling her how he has always wanted to do this, and how he has wanked many times thinking about her. Now he is actually taking her for real. His mouth is eating her cunt, tasting her hot juices as they flow onto the table before his eyes. Lifting his head from her legs he says, "Can I fuck you, Auntie?"

With a huge gasp she screams, "Yes, yes, fuck me hard and fast, and fill me with your lovely hot spunk!" Auntie says she wants to take the hot raw spunk from her nephew right there on the kitchen table.

The plot continues as Auntie becomes pregnant by her nephew, and he continues to stay, fucking her more often than ever. He likes the idea of the baby growing inside her and loves sucking on her huge tits full of milk. This excites them both, and so the phone chat continues over many months.

After many months of implementing these phone chat scenarios, I felt I wanted to do a little bit more. I decided to invest in a web cam, and have a go at putting on a live show like the other girls on the site. I knew it wouldn't be easy for me, as unlike the phone chat, people that booked you were watching you live. This sounded quite demanding, as not only would you have to look good all the time, but also you might only have a short notice of five minutes to be in the right position for the camera. Anyway I decided to give it a go and see how I got on.

Firstly I got all dressed up with all my makeup on, perfect hair in place and wearing a basque etc. I then put the laptop where I could reach it, as you had to write to people at the same time as doing what they asked of you. For instance, when a booking was made, it meant using the computer to accept the booking, and then we both had to complete by exchanging MSN addresses. It all seemed very nerve-racking, and also I had another concern. So far I had only received good ratings on my work and I didn't want to do a poor show and then get given a bad one. A lot of the girls on the site had been given poor ratings for their web cam work, anything from the men complaining about poor lighting, to the girls not doing what they had been asked to do. My biggest setback would be them asking me to walk about or strip for them, when I wasn't able to because of the wheelchair. A few of my regular phone chat men knew I couldn't walk, but most of them didn't as it wasn't necessary for me to tell them unless they were going to visit me for real. In which case, I would always tell them beforehand.

I put a little message on my profile, telling them I was going to be doing a web cam session for approximately two hours, but they must email me before putting in a booking. There I was all dressed up and ready to go, when suddenly the bookings started to flock in; some had read the message about emailing me beforehand and some hadn't. Suddenly I was in a panic, trying to email to each one my circumstances and secondly trying to accept the booking before it timed out. Before I knew it I had accepted my first one.

The camera was on and he was writing to me saying, "Wow, you look lovely." I wrote back thanking him and asked what he would like me to do. He was OK about me not being able to walk and asked me to show him my breasts. I took them out of my basque for him and smiled into the camera. I zoomed the camera right full onto them, rolling them around in my hand, and squeezing my nipples for him. He was writing away. telling me how much he liked them.

I then said, "Would you like to see more of me?"

With that he wrote back saying, "Yes, lie on the bed and open your legs."

At this point I thought, "Oh my God, I hope I can do this gracefully." Somehow I managed to gently lie back, lifting up my skirt, and again directing the light and the camera onto my now wet pussy.

I was very excited at the thought of someone watching me, even though I couldn't see them. The mystery of it did have an element of excitement. Next he said, "Do you have a vibrator handy?" Luckily I had organised all that in advance, just in case I was asked. So I picked it up off the bed and guided it to my mouth, licking the end of it first. I thought a bit of gentle teasing to start with would go down well. I was right, for he wrote telling me he was bursting to come as he had imagined that that was his cock I was sucking. "That was the idea," I thought to myself and it had worked. Next I gently pushed the vibrator between my breasts, as if I was going to tit wank it, again slowly going from my mouth to my tits. I then gently leant right back on the bed opening my legs wide, and just rubbed the tip of the vibrator on to my wet pussy, gently pushing it in and out of me. At the same time I gave him a welcoming smile, as if to say, "I wish this was your hard cock."

The writing from him stopped for a moment. Was he still there, I thought, a bit worried in case he had disappeared through disappointment. Then suddenly the writing came back. "Thanks, that was really good," he wrote. "You made me come for England." Phew, I breathed a sigh of relief. With that we said goodbye and I now had the courage to do the next one.

The next one sadly hadn't read my message about emailing me beforehand, so when the booking came through and I read that he wanted me to parade around the room in stockings and stiletto shoes I had to decline the booking.

The next few went well, pretty much the same as the first one. However, each time I got as nervous as the first in case they didn't like me. Thankfully I continued with the good feedback and didn't pick up any bad ratings for this service. However, I didn't continue to offer this service as I found it too much hard work and very stressful. Also it meant that I had to stay looking perfect all day just in case someone wanted to book me with only a few minutes' notice.

Chapter 28
More Escorting

My confidence was beginning to come back, after Mike's comment. But at first I found it hard believing that men liked coming to see me. It was the next few clients that built me up and made me sure I was worth it.

One of my regular massage customers had spotted me on the escort site. He was delighted to find me there and rang me asking if I would see him for a full personal service and already knowing him made it easier to say yes. I had already been seeing him for about three years and now we were going to go all the way. He turned up much more nervous than the previous times. I was dressed completely differently and his eyes nearly popped out of his head. I had a basque on with my tits bulging out over the top. "Bloody Hell," he commented, "am I looking forward to this," and he went on to tell me he had wanted me from the very first time he had ever met me.

I was shocked as I had not realised, not only did he want to sleep with me for money, but he was asking me out for a real date! I went on to explain that I don't like to mix the two, and having had him as a client it wasn't a good idea. I also had Mike to think about, and I didn't want to go out on a date with other men.

Our hour was sheer pleasure, he knew exactly what to do to turn me on, and his touch was gentle, almost electrifying. I was soon putty in his hands. He whispered in my ear that he loved me, although I was sure this was not true. However, it did the trick for me at the time, and I came like Niagara Falls. He left very satisfied and he still continues to call for regular visits. He gave me back my confidence in escorting and I now knew I was to put the old self back on and get in the saddle.

Some days I would feel like Mrs Doubtfire, changing from one outfit to another. Some men liked me dressed as a tart in all the gear, and others would like me completely naked. Then there were the ones who like uniforms. I have a couple of different nurses' uniforms, dark blue with a white stripe, and the other all white. This went down well with the clients; a naughty nurse wearing a white bra underneath and no panties worked a treat. I had other outfits, like a leather bra that had holes where your breasts should be, so they just kind of hung out. Long black silky gloves, or short net gloves … men loved it all. I also had to keep changing the photos on my site, so that it would keep them interested. I had got permission from some of my clients to take some naughty pictures whilst they were fucking me. It was difficult to do and good fun at times, as I had to hold the camera with one hand as they were fucking me. They got extremely turned on by this, knowing they were going to be pictured fucking me on my site. I kept their faces out for obvious reasons, although one or two said I could use their face shot when they were giving me oral sex.It was clear I had mastered the art of most positions on the bed even though I was wheelchair-bound.

Escorting had its down-sides, one of them being that you were booked and obliged to provide a full personal service without even knowing what the person looked like. It was not a case of picking the right man, it was a case of judging by the sound of their voice as to whether you would accept them or not. I more often than not went with my instinct. If I wasn't sure of their attitude over the phone, I simply said I was busy.

I would always get ready feeling anxious. What if they were awful and dirty, or they walked in and didn't like me, although thankfully that never ever happened with the escorting. I would try to get a feel over the phone for what they liked, as I felt it was useless trying to work it out when they were here. For instance, if they wanted lots of oral, there would be no point in trying to shove my tits in their face. If they liked it hard, I didn't want to waste time doing it gently. I also found this helped them get turned on before the visit, as I knew from experience that once they have booked a girl, they then like to fantasise about what they would like to do with them.

One particular day I had to meet a man with a very large frame, standing over six feet tall and very muscular. He had a hairy chest and was very manly. He said, "I have a question to ask you."

"What is that?" I replied.

"Can I wear stockings and suspenders whilst I'm with you?" he said.

I looked at him and panicked a little, thinking, "I don't have anything to fit you." I smiled and said, "Yes, of course," and with that he started to pull his trousers down, revealing a black and pink suspender belt and black stockings. He stood there looking at me, waiting for my reaction.

I looked enthusiastic and said, "OK, that's great, you look fantastic." He obviously liked what I said, as he was starting to get very aroused by the whole situation. He then asked if I would take some photos of him sitting around dressed like this and again I obliged. His next desire was to actually fuck me dressed like this. Again I responded eagerly, trying not to spoil his fun, and we got onto the bed. All the time I was praising him, and telling him how sexy and slutty he looked, and this continued as he entered me. Getting more and more turned on, he finally shot his load. After he thanked me, he said that he had always had a fantasy about fucking someone dressed like this, but his wife would have been horrified. To me it was just another day at the office.

Another client would always text me before an appointment; he never calls, just texts, to see if I am available and also for me to tell him what I am going to do with him when he arrives. He likes me to be waiting for him, lying on the bed naked, wrapped in only a fur blanket. I am also instructed to start to play with myself before he gets to me, so I am nice and wet for him. He then walks in and sits on the bed, and slowly unwraps me out of the blanket, while caressing me from head to toe. He does this gently and carefully which makes me tingle all over. He likes to see me get so turned on, and talking nicely to me he glides his hand down my body until it is touching and stroking my wet pussy. He tells me how he wants to make me come so badly for him. By now I am putty in his hands and begging him to fuck me.

He proceeds to stand up and undress for me. I watch him strip off his clothes, showing me his hard cock. Then he gets a little more dominant; climbing onto the bed, he positions himself into a "sixty-nine" while licking and sucking me. He loves to please me and will do any command I give him. We even play a little game where he will pretend to be cross with me for being naughty, and for that he puts his hand over my neck and calls me names, all of which I love so much. I have built up a trust with him, and I know that he would stop if I didn't like it.

As he fucks me he goes from one personality to the other, fucking every way he can. One minute he is cross with me, the next he is telling me he loves me. Between the two different scenarios I am so excited that I feel I should be paying him. He comes very easily, as seeing me so excited is always just too much for him, and often we both manage to climax at the same time. One day he arrived with a lot of presents for me, various vibrators and gadgets that he could use to pleasure me on different occasions. He is now one of my regulars and has got to know what I like.

One day another rather unusual client took me by surprise. I had known him a few years through the massaging. He then found I did escorting through the website, and asked if he could see me. I accepted and thought it would be easier as I knew him already. I was so wrong; although I knew him I didn't know his sexual fantasies, and by God did he shock me. He asked if I liked to be dominated. This was something that I never usually offered and I thought the girls that do offer it must be very brave. You never knew who would turn up or if they would hurt you, or even try to kill you. Anyway I said I hadn't really done it much, only in playing around a little, but because I knew him I would allow him to do it. He started off not too bad, but seemed to get rougher and harder by the second as he got more excited.

We went to the bedroom and he pinned me on the bed really hard, which is not something I would usually worry about too much, but I could see he was wanting to get even rougher still. He spun me over on top of him and started to call me names in the process, slapping my tits as hard as he could. He was slapping both of them and trying to bite me. I still had an element of doubt, but again as I knew him I kept telling myself he wouldn't dare do anything too major to hurt me.

After a really hard fucking and bashing in the bedroom he ordered me to put my face down on the bed. He put his hand over the back of my neck, holding me down with my face to one side. He told me he was going to wank himself off over my pretty little face. I was kind of glad as I thought that if he came, he would then calm down, as I was not sure how much more I could take. He soon came over my face as he had promised and I felt relieved it was all over. I didn't enjoy it one bit, and decided I would never repeat being a "Sub" for a client. The next day my tits were bruised and sore, and after that experience I told him I was sorry but I didn't want to see him again. I am sure he didn't mean any harm, and understood when I told him how I felt, but that is not one of my services to be repeated.

A good experience for me was when I met a lady one day when out shopping, and we became good friends. I told her about my escorting and she decided to give it a try. We lived fairly near to each other and she asked if we could do some clients together. She said to just call and we could meet up.

This particular day one of my regular massage clients was with me and we were talking about a two-girl thing. He said he really would love it. I had never offered him a full personal before, and explained that I still didn't feel happy about going any further with him myself. However my friend would like to come around and help if I called her. He agreed eagerly and she arrived within a few minutes. We were both sides of him, touching him and teasing. I asked if he would like her to take her clothes off. He nodded yes, so she took off her dress, and just stood there in her bra and knickers. I then asked if he would like to kiss her and touch her breasts. I watched as this happened and I then asked if he would like to lick her pussy. So removing her panties and turning her round he knelt down in front of me and started to lick her juicy wet pussy. Then I suggested that he should fuck her and again he nodded. I took a condom, placed it over his cock and guided it into her as far as it would go up. As he fucked her I played with her nipples and talked to them both, giving them one almighty orgasm. "Wow," he said, "I think it must be all my birthdays and Christmases in one."

Chapter 29
Overnight Bookings

I had also offered, like the other girls on the site, to do an overnight service. I would go and stay with a man at a hotel room for the evening and sleep there for the night; that is, if there was any sleep to be had.

The first booking came through and I was beside myself with worry, not knowing what the hell I would have to do for the whole night long. I had put an offer on the site advertising a half price deal, since at the time I needed the money and was grateful for the booking. The next question was would they turn up or let me down. Well I was lucky as he kept in contact with text messages throughout the day. I turned up wearing the same things as I had shown in the pictures on my website, including the blond wig, basque and stockings. He shook my hand and introduced himself. He had fair hair, stocky build, and a pleasant happy face. I think he could tell I was nervous, as he had a bottle of wine open on the side and offered me one. "I don't usually," I said, but I did on this occasion, grabbing the glass and gulping it down.

We sat and talked for a while, he was chatty and so that helped as he took the lead in the conversation. After an hour of talking he suggested having a relaxing bath. That's great, I thought, as that will take up a bit of time. I was praying he didn't want me to join him in the bath as I would not have felt very comfortable about this. If I had the perfect figure, things would have been very different, but looking as I did with scars from my previous operations, I felt I would rather keep as much of my clothes on as possible for now. He was fine and didn't expect me to get in. I sat on the edge of the bath, running soapy water down his chest, and talking to him naughtily. I asked him what his biggest fantasy was, and what was the most outrageous thing he had ever done etc.

This kind of talk began to turn him on and after his bath he wanted to waste no time in shoving his hard cock into my mouth. We started in the bathroom and then he picked me up out of my wheelchair and placed me on the bed. Kneeling over my face he looked down at me as he practically forced his huge cock down my throat until he shot his load. "Thanks," he said, "that was great."

I sat up, pulled my clothes back into place and watched him light up a cigarette. "Would you like one?" he said.

"Oh no," I replied, "I don't smoke."

He asked why I had some pictures on the site of me smoking and I explained that it was for the purpose of the photos only. Some men had requested I take some smoking pictures as they like to see a woman holding a cigarette and blowing smoke.

"I can pretend to smoke for you now if you'd like me to," I said.

"No, it's not a problem," he replied, "I'm not bothered either way."

We talked some more and not too long after, he started to feel hard again. This time I climbed on top of him and teased him a while, kissing his face off and talking dirty. He rolled me over, tearing away at my clothes frantically and pulling my tits out. Next he was fucking me in every position, moaning and thrusting like mad until again he shot his load. I remember looking at the clock and noticing that it was now just after midnight. I thought to myself, "Will I be getting any sleep or will I just be fucked the whole night through?"

He suggested we get into bed. Great, I thought, we are going to sleep, but no, I was wrong. He cuddled me so tight and wanted to talk for hours. We were just relaxing and I started to nod off when he woke me up, saying, "Suck my cock for me again." So I did, and like the last time he shot his load into my mouth. Not long after that he did eventually fall asleep. I was looking at him, thinking, "This is not Mike," as it did feel strange being next to someone else as they slept. The next thing I remember was being woken up again with him kneeling over me and begging me to suck him off yet again. It was now six o'clock in the morning and he had to leave. We said goodbye and I fell asleep, worn out from my hard night's work. That was my first overnight and although he was a lovely man, I found it very stressful and demanding. I hoped if I had another one it would be slightly easier.

The second overnight came a few weeks later, and again I had an offer on reducing the price. The booking came through and we spoke on the phone for a while, arranging when he would be able to come down. He was due to stay overnight in the area and he wanted me to stay the night at his hotel. We had arranged to meet in the restaurant about seven, and he was there waiting for me with a huge smile and a strong handshake. He greeted me and directed me over to the table. He was in his early fifties, greying hair, medium build and he had a gentle pleasant manner about him. I had asked him over the phone what his favourite colour was and he told me red, so I offered to wear a red low cut top and skirt. This top showed him a good bulging cleavage as we sat across the candle-lit table, talking. I dared him to put his hand on my leg, he laughed and said, "You are something else," but taking me up on the dare he did it. I told him how good that felt, and looking around the restaurant to see if anyone was looking, I asked if he would dare brush his hand over my tits as he stood up. Again he took up the challenge and did just that. "Let's not waste any more time," he said, rushing me back to his room.

He barely waited to get the door shut before starting to undress me. He said, "Now that I've been looking at you all evening through your clothes, I want to take them all off."

I gulped and thought, "Oh no, what if he doesn't like my body, I don't, so why should he?" But there was no stopping him, he was undoing every hook on my basque and every button on my skirt, and next I was lying on the bed in front of him completely naked.

"That's better," he said.

"Really?" I thought, as I was surprised.

He said, "I prefer to see a woman's naked body," as he was stepping out of his clothes. I looked at his penis and it was hard as a rock, so I figured my naked body had not been as bad for him as I had first thought.

He continued to open my legs and give me one hell of an oral session, licking and sucking my juicy wet pussy for about half an hour. This was such a turn on and by now I was about ready for anything. He asked me at this point if I could dominate him a little, and tell him exactly what I wanted him to do. I made him lie on back on the bed with his arms and legs spread wide. I asked him to shut his eyes as I started to pull and suck on his nipples as hard as I could without hurting him. I then made him roll over onto his tummy and spanked his arse as hard as I could. He was really loving it, and on the verge of coming. I told him he wasn't allowed to come just yet, and I made him wait, although I still kept him right on the brink. Finally I climbed on top of him and pushed his cock into me, shouting, "Go on, give it to me now!" He had a massive climax and was shaking all over with pleasure.

He had bought a bottle of wine, although we hadn't opened it yet, as after all the teasing in the restaurant he had forgotten all about it. We sat and had a drink and talked for a few hours, and then he suggested we get some sleep. I was so relieved to hear that he wanted to sleep, especially after what had happened on the first overnight. I can't tell you how nice it was to only work for a few hours and then go to sleep. In the morning he crept out of bed, and although I was awake I pretended to still be asleep. He left without disturbing me.

Chapter 30
Overnight with Mike

Things at Mike's home were getting tricky and some questions were being asked. Mike also wanted a little more freedom, although he had always had a lot, and had very much done as he had liked for the past 18 years. His family had been away again, leaving him free all weekend. Mike and Colin were going fishing. Mike had not been before and wasn't too sure if he was going to like it, but thought it would be relaxing anyway. When the Saturday came I had a really bad migraine, so the fishing was abandoned and Mike stayed with me, massaging my neck. I had never seen him so calm before, totally relaxed. That evening Mike, Colin and I had a meal and watched television. Mike went home at midnight.

The next day Mike spent the day with me again before his family came back. His partner was a very strong woman, who didn't expect Mike to have a life outside of her control. He could not have said to her, "I've made some friends, and would like to go round for a meal." She could do whatever she wanted, had many, many friends and expected Mike to tag along to every party or gathering that she arranged. If he wanted to do something else, he was questioned either by his partner or his daughter (although only after she found out about us). I said to him why don't you arrange for us all to meet somehow.

We arranged it with some imaginary story about him knowing me from meeting me outside PC World. My chair had broken down and he had helped me to get home. He told her this, as we accidentally on purpose arranged to meet at the local restaurant.

Then he introduced Colin and me to his family. Well, only his son in the end as his daughter had made other arrangements. I don't think she ever believed Mike's story. On the way home she said she wasn't sure about me. Perhaps you could call it women's instinct. She was right, and we were wrong to have ever believed it. It didn't end there, however, as his daughter liked to sing and I was very interested in her as I loved it too. I had all the recording equipment and wanted to meet her and hear her voice.

They did agree to this and Mike, his partner and daughter came along for one evening of singing. I thought it went well and the daughter seemed to enjoy the attention. She even drove back home at one point to fetch her own microphone and some songs she had written. If that evening had gone to plan, I had decided that Mike and I would only be friends from that moment and would not sleep with each other again. I didn't want or plan to cheat on his family, he had pursued me. All I wanted was to put this behind me, and for us all to be friends.

Mike had a swimming pool and hot tub at his house, he was desperate for me to go around there and enjoy it. That evening he suggested it to his partner and she looked a little horrified, but didn't rule it out. They all left and I waited to hear from Mike the next day with the result. He said she was very quiet on the way home. I was sure then it wasn't going to work, even for us to be friends. I told him it had to stop but he didn't agree and I became angry. I was thinking I can't do this to your family, they don't like me, and how can we now even be friends. Mike was still not ready to give up, and insisted we try and call to say it was nice having them over and also we would like to take them up on the offer of the hot tub. This was the last chance. She had at that point accepted when Mike said about us coming over. However, that day it thundered really badly. I didn't want to go, and she certainly didn't want us to come.

However, Mike insisted again, even getting it hot when he arrived home from work. What I hadn't realised was that they had had a huge row before we arrived, and she had walked out. I couldn't understand why just Mike was there, with his son upstairs the whole evening, staying out of the way. We finished in the hot tub, and went into the house at about 10.45. I kept asking Mike where she was, and just as we were leaving he said they had fallen out over us going over. I did feel awkward and upset for him trying so hard. However, I felt guilty to have caused the family problems. When I didn't know these things it was very different as I could just see Mike as another unhappy client, with needs that were not satisfied. Now I had met all his family and they were real people with feelings. I wasn't proud of myself, and I wished it would all just go away. Things were very strained between me and Mike after that. He kept ringing me and begging to see me. I kept avoiding him. I suppose I was hoping he would put his family first. But was it too late?

As I said previously, the adult site I was on also offered a phone chat service which I did a lot. I didn't do a lot of escorting at this time, as I was very careful. If I didn't like the sound of them or they were too young I would say no. I had built up a few regulars and between the phone chat service and the massaging, I was able to get by on the money. Mike would get very frustrated, as often he would ring me, and because I was busy, he was not able to get hold of me. This would frustrate him so much. I was also trying to get my head around the disaster with his family. I would contemplate if I should just let him go and make it work with his family.

One day he wrote me a horrible email, saying, "Do I have to book you like one of your clients just to talk to you?" This email came on a bad day, as I was going to the hospital to get my results. On reading this I was so angry. "Why today?" I asked myself. Did he not have any regard for the fact that I was worried? I went off to the hospital with steam coming out of my ears. I thought I would calm down, but this time I didn't. When I got back I wrote him an email and said that's it, he had pushed me too far. The hospital had done some test and I was feeling awful, and this was one big mess. With Mike giving me grief and not feeling well, yet still trying to work, I wasn't sure how much more I could take.

My health was going through a real bad spell. After going

to Mike's house a week ago and using the hot tub, I started to feel really ill. I was getting terrible headaches, I had pains down my legs, I was very weak, and generally very much under the weather. I took no notice at first, just trying to carry on, but in the end I couldn't get out of bed or eat. This went on for three weeks. In the meantime I wasn't able to cope with Mike so I had no contact at all. He would ring, email or text Colin to see how I was. I would receive emails from him, but didn't reply. I just couldn't be bothered with all the hassle, feeling guilty towards his family and feeling ill at the same time.

I found it easy to cut Mike off at this point and I would have stuck to it if Colin had not kept on and on relaying messages back to me on how he was. He would write to me saying how he needed me, and telling me how he wasn't able to eat. All his work colleagues had noticed, and one had asked if he was ill. The only people not to have noticed were his family, none of them. He had lost stones, he had not been eating his dinners in the evening and yet they never noticed. Eventually one day his partner did make a remark and said, "Are you ill?"

Mike continued to try to help me even though I wasn't at that point there for him. He would continue to talk to Colin, asking what I was able to eat. Every few days he would drop a food parcel in for me, consisting of freshly squeezed orange juice, strawberries, cream cakes, and anything he could think of. I was grateful, but also found it irritating as I wondered if it was genuine or if he was trying to buy me back. I asked Colin to tell him to stop, but he didn't listen and continued the kindness for weeks.

Colin would look after me, and eventually I agreed to visit the doctor who tested me for several things including Glandular Fever. A few days later the result came back and I was told I had an inflamed liver, which explained all the symptoms I had been suffering. I was relieved as never had I felt so ill for so long, Mike at times hadn't believed me, and thought I was just saying it to get off the hook for not bothering with him. Colin on the other hand was getting more and more worried as he had never seen me like this before. Eventually after the third week I started to feel a lot better. My appetite came back, and the terrible headaches had subsided.

I was told by Colin that Mike in the meantime was worried about possibly facing redundancy. I did feel for him, but also knew if I contacted him it would mean getting involved and ending up back where we were before. This particular week Colin told me that Mike's family were away, leaving him alone. He kept asking Colin if we could all go out for a meal. In turn Colin repeatedly asked me, as he didn't know what to tell Mike. I think Colin really felt for Mike at this point, he felt in the middle, wanting to help him but at the same time not wanting to put too much pressure on me. In the end I decided I would agree to go out for a meal with Mike, but wanted it to be at the end of the week, so he couldn't pressurise me too much. I knew if he was on his own he would want to ring me, or keep calling round. I agreed the Friday evening would be OK. Colin and I turned up at the arranged time and all arrangements had been done between the two of them. I still had not spoken to Mike directly.

We arrived at the restaurant and I felt at first very hostile towards him. Although I tried to act normal I was failing miserably. Mike looked so pleased to see me, but with such sadness in his face at my hostility. He looked very thin and drawn and after a while I couldn't keep up my bad feelings towards him any longer. That was the problem with Mike. Whenever he upset me I could be strong and remain mad over the phone, but as soon as I saw him I would feel sad at hurting him, and give in.

The evening started to improve and Mike and I started to talk normally, as we always did, and before long we were laughing. He was telling me his worries over the redundancy at work. I kept trying to reassure him, telling him it wouldn't be him. After the meal he insisted on paying for us, saying he wanted to.

Normally Mike would not be out late, but whilst in the restaurant he had told me he had joined the local casino. Not to gamble, as he is far from a gambling man. He had only joined because I was a member, and he wanted to just turn up there one night and surprise me. I was surprised at this, made a joke of it and suggested we could pop in there for an hour now. He jumped at this (probably as it meant he could be with me longer), although in actual fact we only stayed for a while. Mike seemed very happy and it was about 12.30 am when we went back down the road towards the cars. He was laughing, saying how his partner would die if she could see him now, out at this time of the morning, when usually he would be tucked up in bed by 10 pm. I think this was always a sore point between the two of them, as she was always up late, out with friends, and he would go to bed so early. We all found it funny. Saying goodbye next to the cars, we thanked him for a lovely evening. I apologised for not being there for him lately and promised I would be now. We waved each other off at the roundabout, he went his way and we went ours.

On the way home I said to Colin that I had felt guilty for not being there for Mike. After seeing him it made me realise that no matter what his family thought I had to carry on seeing and being there for him. It was true what he had told me about not being able to eat. He had lost a lot of weight and perhaps, I thought, he really did need me in his life.

The very next day the emails were flowing in as before, thanking me for being there in his life again. This time I replied without hesitation. Colin was so happy we had got back to normal. He said Mike was such a good person, I must look after him. I had to agree as I considered him reliable, kind, and thoughtful. That was a major turning point in our relationship.

One thing that did shock me was that Mike had told me he had taken a woman out at work a few times in his lunch breaks. He said he did it to try and get over me, reassuring me it was nothing more than kissing and cuddling. He said he thought we were over. I tried to see it from his point of view at the time, and reminded him that even if he wasn't with me, it seemed he would still be seeking love from another woman. This was dangerous and confirmed to me that whatever happened between us, his relationship with his partner looked very doubtful. He said the woman at work had paid him a lot of attention. It worried me what his intentions would be towards her now, as they had got close through the redundancy problem. It was drawing to the end of September when the big decision at work would be made.

Just before the final outcome Mike had been asked to go to Amsterdam on a trip with his work, for two days. I said I had always wanted to go there. "Really?" he said and within a few minutes we were looking on the internet at the flight prices. There was a deal on, where you could fly return for about £35. He didn't hesitate and booked two more flight tickets for Colin and me to go with him. Mike had for as long as I can remember wanted to spend the entire night with me. This was something I offered on the adult website I was on. I had only ever done one up to now, and Mike hated it. Here was his big chance. "Can I sleep with you for the night?" he asked. I said I would ask Colin. He didn't mind, so it was all arranged.

Colin had to come as it was impossible for Mike to take me to another country without the help of Colin. Mike had never really pushed the wheelchair outside, let alone tried to manage on a flight, taxis and whatever help I might need. Mike was happy, as he was so excited at the thought of having me all night long. So two rooms were booked and I was to stay with Mike in his room. Colin didn't mind as long as we were all getting along and happy.

Mike didn't tell his partner until two days before, just in case she had suggested going with him, although she hadn't done before when he had to go away on business. But he didn't want to take a chance. She accepted it but did say, "Why didn't you tell me before?"

The day was all set and emails were flying back and forth throughout the day. We were to meet Mike at 5 pm at the local airport. Bags packed and all excited, we pulled into the car park at the same time. We left the cars and booked in for our flight. I hadn't been away for a while so I was so happy to be going on this trip.

We had a nice flight, landed at about 9.30 pm, and then caught a coach to our hotel. At this point Mike wasn't sure if he would still be allowed to sleep with me all night or not. Colin and I had discussed it and so with Colin's permission we thought we would surprise Mike at the hotel. We had a nice meal, and as it was getting late, Mike asked, "Well, do I get to keep you for the night?"

Colin and I smiled and said, "Of course you do." Mike was like a little kid, full of excitement, and rushed me back to the room. We said goodnight to Colin who was in the room opposite.

Mike had told me previously of all the things he wanted to do if he was allowed to keep me for the night. One thing he wanted was for me to bath him, as this was something I really enjoyed doing. I ran him a nice hot bath, and sat beside him, gently swishing the hot soapy water over his chest, and gently rubbing it. I tried to give him lots of tender loving care and make him feel so special. I even dried him, covered him with talc and brushed his hair.

His next wish was for me to take my bra off and go around the room topless for him for a while. He was getting more excited and kept saying, "I just can't believe I have you all to myself all night long." He said he was obsessed with looking at my profile on the adult website. He would read every word I had written over and over again, studying each and every photo in great detail. He said that it was like looking into a window of my life, and he would watch the changes I used to make every day. He said how he would get so jealous of the other men that I would see, and yet get extremely turned on thinking about me being naughty. It got to about 2 am and there was no sign of us sleeping. Mike had one thing on his mind, and that was not to waste one second of this night. This was a very special night and I joked with him, saying how much it would have cost if he had been a proper overnight booking.

It got to about 4 am and we were both very tired as it had been a long day, but neither of us could sleep. We lay there cuddling and talking. Mike had to be up at 5.30 to be at the other side of Amsterdam for about 8 am. We kept saying we must go to sleep or we would feel like zombies later, and then we would start to joke with each other and laugh again. We said OK, let's strike a deal. If we lie here for ten minutes quiet, that will give either one of us the chance to drop off to sleep, and if this happens we mustn't wake the other one up.

The next thing I remember was Mike sitting on my side of the bed in his suit, leaning over me saying goodbye. I had been the one to fall asleep first and I hadn't even heard him get ready. He said he would ring me later when he had finished the job he had to do.

I didn't go back to sleep, as I needed to make sure Colin was OK. He was fine, and we got ready and went down to breakfast together. Colin asked me if Mike was OK and I said he was very happy. Colin and I had a wonderful understanding of the situation. He didn't have any problems with Mike and me, and I trusted Colin's honesty about it. We had spent many hours over the last few months discussing my job, and my relationship with Mike, the whole lot. Colin's attitude was so totally unselfish of his own feelings. He wanted me more than anything in the world to be happy. He always feared that should something happen to him, I would not have anyone there for me. I don't think people to this day really understand our relationship, or how he is able to share me with others. All I can say is after seventeen years of being together, he knows and understands me more than anyone ever could. He wants me to be happy, treated right, and taken care of.

After breakfast we settled the last minute billing and waited for the phone call from Mike to say he was on his way back. We had arranged to meet him back at the railway station, as we wanted to go into the centre and all look around together.

Mike called just after 12 and so we got the coach to the station and met him. It was a glorious sunny day, not too hot and not at all cold. We had to get the train into Amsterdam centre. This all went very smoothly, and they both lifted the chair together onto the train. We all had one big ambition whilst we were in Amsterdam and that was to go and look at the famous red light district. I was as curious as the men as after all I wanted to see the competition. We asked several friendly people for directions and we were directed down this street and that street, until eventually we found it.

There were all these beautiful woman sitting there in glass windows, for the entire world to see. They were wearing sexy underwear and offering their services. I felt envious of their beautiful bodies and faces, but I kept remembering there is always someone for everyone. I had also learnt from my own experience that not all men like the young perfect-looking woman who coldly takes your money. Most men want to have a girlfriend experience. I figured I must have come somewhere in between or clients would not have come back to me. So I kept a positive attitude, and smiled nicely at the girls as we went past. I sniggered to myself that they had no idea I was in the same business. Mike and Colin were fascinated and I asked if either would like to pay one a visit, but they both declined. So we just had a good laugh looking, going into the sex shops and soaking up the atmosphere. After a while we decided to stop off at a café and have a drink outside in the sunshine. We sat there chatting, laughing and getting on so well.

Our flight home wasn't until late that evening. Mike and I had started to lose the plot a bit due to our lack of sleep the night before. We tried drinking coffee but we were both getting so tired, it was hard to keep it together. We both joked and said it was a good job we weren't there for two nights, as the second one would have been sleeping only. At last the flight home came, and we arrived back in England safe. Saying goodbye to Mike at that point was hard, as I had just had the best two days I could think of in a long time. I was truly grateful and enjoyed every second of our little overnight together. It had been a huge turning point for us all. Mike had to now return home to his family. It was hard to let him go.

Chapter 31
More Trips

The next morning I woke up to a lovely warm email from Mike telling me how much he had enjoyed being with me for the night and how he had missed not waking up to me that morning. He said he was hoping for some more trips to come up so we could be together again. It was only a few days later he suggested taking a day's holiday from work so that we could have a day out somewhere together. We decided to go to Beaulieu. It wasn't so much the place, but the time to be together.

He picked me up early that morning and we set off with the radio blasting out great songs. We sang along to them as we went along the country roads. We seemed to be able to chat away about anything. I was always interested in what he had to say, and he likewise. We talked a lot about our pasts, and we also discussed Mike's future. He had been a little upset a few days before, as his partner had been leaning over the table, accidentally revealing her cleavage to him. When she saw him looking, she gave him a dirty look, and immediately pulled her top up as if to say, "What are you looking at?" This upset him a lot as not only did she never pay him any attention, but if he was caught paying her some, she reacted with even more rejection.

We had a lovely day, followed by a nice meal in a pub. Mike was getting some looks in the pub as he clearly was all over me, holding my hand and looking into my eyes. We thought we had better make a move before we got thrown out for doing things in public. We joked about stopping off in the New Forest on the way home for a fuck. This didn't stay a joke for very long and before we knew it, we were parked up in the middle of the forest under some trees. I was there with my top down and my legs on the dashboard. Neither of us seemed to care at that point. It was so horny being out there in the broad daylight having a sexual encounter. We were both like a couple of starved rabbits trying to fit everything in. Eventually we thought we had better go back as it was getting late. Mike had to pretend he had been at work. He dropped me off, stayed about half an hour and then went home, but continued to write or text me all evening.

The next few days again brought some great news Mike had been given a trip to Ipswich, with his work. It was just a very small job for him to perform, but as it was such a long way, it meant staying overnight in a hotel. He rang me all excited and asking if I would like to go. "Of course I would," I said. So on the Wednesday we were off again in a hire car driving happily up the motorway, singing and laughing to the songs on the radio.

I am very naughty at times, and while on the M25 these two blokes drove past us in a white van. They glanced over and smiled as I had a rather low cut top on as usual and showing a rather good cleavage. This is something I am very well known for. Mike spotted them, and he was encouraging me to tease them. Laughing, I smiled back at them. This went on for a few miles, with the white van weaving in and out of traffic to keep up with us. I said to Mike, perhaps you had better lose them or they may think we really would like them to follow us. He agreed and luckily they turned off at the next exit. We were now nearly at Colchester, where we were going to stay as there were no rooms available in Ipswich.

As soon as we got to the room Mike took me to bed and our clothes were flung everywhere. We made love and cuddled before going to the restaurant for a nice evening meal. We were very happy. Mike said how much he loved me and said he was falling deeper and deeper for me. I also had started to love him as he was beginning to really become part of my life. I guess after all this time I had finally let him right into my world, which was not something I did very easily.

Coming home we listened to the radio or talked, it didn't

really matter by now. We had got to the point were you don't feel awkward if there is a silence between you. We were both happy, we liked the same music, and we could talk about anything.

On returning home we called Colin to see if he wanted to come with us for a meal at the Casino. We were due a complimentary one and I had promised Mike we would take him for being so good to us. He had just this one evening left before he had to go home to his family again. We had the meal, and I said, "Could I borrow just £20 to put in a fruit machine?" Mike had big issues about this. He hated gambling, and tried to stop me, but I joked and said I would do it anyway. I put the £20 in the machine and within a few seconds had won £200. Mike was so shocked. I took the money out and split it between the three of us. We left the Casino a bit richer and very happy after another great couple of days. We again waved goodbye to Mike as he set off for home.

Chapter 32
Breaking Up

All the latest activity between Mike and me had masked some of the reality that was happening at his work, as the big dread of redundancy was still lurking there in the background with only a few days now until the results. The Big day was the Friday. I remember it well as I decided not to take any work, but to be here for Mike in case he was in a state and needed me. Plus I couldn't concentrate as it was in my mind as much as it could be. After all, if Mike was upset by something now, it had an immediate impact on me also, as he was so much part of my life.

That Friday, like all the others, he left work at 12.30 and got to me about 1 pm. When he walked in I asked what had happened, and he said about twenty had been laid off but not him. I was so relieved for him. I wanted to share his afternoon after so much worry and to be there to enjoy his relief as well. However, this was not meant to be, as a few minutes after he told me, his mobile rang, and it was his partner. She said she had a problem at her work and wanted him to go up there and fix something. Without any hesitation he said, "All right, I'll be there in about 15 minutes."

I looked at him totally shocked. "Mike," I said, "you can't just go. I've taken the day off to be here for you. Now you're going to just leave me and carry on as if nothing was wrong." I had lost money to be there for him, and turned down some of my regulars. Yet here he was saying, "I've got to go."

Just before he left he hit me with another shocking statement. He asked if I would have a problem with him taking out the woman from work. The woman he had seen in the summer when I wasn't there for him. He said, "Do you mind if I take her for a drink?" as they wanted to talk about the redundancies. He said she had asked him if they could go out and talk somewhere.

I was totally taken back. Without wanting to sound as if I thought I owned him or anything, I said, "Do what you like." He again asked if I had a problem. At this point I was fuming.

"Do I have a problem?" I said. "How can I not have a problem when you were kissing her face off just a few months ago? But after all, if you really need to go out with her then don't let me stop you."

I think he got my point and said, "I won't go if you are not happy about it." He then had to leave as he had told his partner he would be only 15 minutes and half an hour had passed. He left saying, "I'll try and come back later, if I can get away," but never did.

A good few days passed, and the only contact we had was via emails. The following Friday he did a bit of shopping for me, and called in to see me in the afternoon. I hadn't been too good and had suffered a bad spell of headaches. I think it was all the stress, and not knowing what was happening with Mike. I was upset as I had tried so hard to be there for him throughout the redundancy scare. I had taken days off and always tried to answer the phone when he rang. However my finances had suffered over the last few weeks due to not working every hour I could to pay the bills.

Mike and I discussed this and he understood it was partly his fault that I hadn't worked. He offered to try and help me as the stress of money was becoming a vicious circle. The more I worried the more I suffered with bad migraines, and then was unable to work. The following Friday Mike said he would help me by lending me £500 towards what I had lost. He couldn't stay as his son needed him to be somewhere and Mike had to take him. Mike called in really quick offering me a cheque. He then said, "If I make it out for £600, do you have a hundred in cash on you, as I am in a rush and it will save me drawing it out of the wall." I agreed and handed him the hundred pounds and thanked him sincerely for the cheque. He left immediately to meet his son. I couldn't do anything with the cheque, as it was 3.30 on a Friday and the banks wouldn't clear it until the following week anyway. So I breathed a sigh of relief, looking at the £600 cheque. I was worried as I was a hundred down in actual cash, but knew I would get it back after a few days.

Things at Mike's house had been coming to a head. The pair of them had been saying they were going to have a talk, which she had put off several times. I kept telling him he needed to sort things out and tell her the truth. He agreed but felt worried. They had said for the past week we will talk tomorrow, but it never happened. It was finally planned for Saturday the 23rd of October. A day after Mike had written me that cheque. On the Saturday, in the afternoon, Mike, knowing he was having a big heart to heart with her that evening, came over to us and helped us do a big food shop. I paid for it all, Mike just helped us in the supermarket and then when we got back home to put it all away. He seemed a little worried and distant. I wasn't surprised; I knew he didn't like confrontation and dreaded the ordeal he had to face later that evening.

He left us, said goodbye and drove home. I was so worried about him, not knowing how it would all go. I waited patiently by the computer for any emails, but heard nothing. That night I didn't sleep for worry about how things would go. The next morning he wrote an email saying it hadn't happened. After all that stress, it hadn't even happened. He in the end had told her they would need to talk today, which was the 24th of October. He said in the email he was going to talk to her at eleven o'clock when he took her up a cup of tea. I wrote back fast before he went offline, wishing him good luck and reminding him I loved him. I also said I would be there for him however it went.

I kept looking at the clock. Eleven came, my heart was in my mouth for Mike, and also for me, hoping he could be strong. The way things had gone for him at home lately were really bad. She had been growing more suspicious of his behaviour and suspected he was up to something. He had changed his pattern, leaving home earlier in the mornings and returning later at night. Not that it made much difference as she was more often out than in when he arrived home. He did most of the cooking for the family, and she even complained if the dinner wasn't on the table when she eventually did get home. This was often late as he used to ring me whilst he was waiting for her or the kids to come home. This used to be nearly every evening.

The day was a very long one and all I did was look at the time. It got to 9 pm before I heard another thing. Then I had an email and I read it with my heart in my mouth. They had finally talked and it was not looking good at all. She had just popped out for a few minutes to drop their son somewhere, giving him a chance to write to me quickly. The emails were flying back and forth as fast as we could before she came home and caught him. He said for the last ten hours she had been going absolutely mental at him, screaming and shouting. He said he was worn out with it all; it was getting near to his bed time, and all he wanted was to just stop now and go to bed. He said she was getting very nasty. I was so worried and I told him maybe he should walk out if she got too angry, so as not to inflame her even more. She now knew all about me. Ten o'clock came and went, which was Mike's normal bed time. He had been in the habit of text messaging me every night at this time when he was in bed to say goodnight to me. Telling me he loved and missed me. It was a little routine we had adopted over the last few months. So when it came to ten I wasn't sure if he had escaped her bile and anger towards him, or whether he had managed to go to bed or not. I didn't get a text message – not at ten and not in fact for a very long time.

The last time I had heard from Mike was at 9 pm on Sunday the 24th of October 2005. By Monday I was thinking, "I know he'll contact me today, as he will be desperate to tell me how things are." But nothing – no email, no text, not even a phone call. I was beside myself with worry. I wasn't even sure if he was alright. He didn't seem it; in his last emails, he seemed scared.

Not knowing what to do, and out of desperation, Colin rang his landline. She answered the phone. Colin asked for Mike and she just slammed the phone down. It had not solved anything. If Mike had answered, at least we would have known he was safe and well. Then Colin tried ringing Mike's work. They said he was off for a few days. Nothing seemed to make any sense. I knew he was going through a difficult nightmare, but thought he would contact me somehow even to say he was all right – or not, as the case may be.

The cheque he had given me on the previous Friday had to be put in the bank on the Monday, as I was so desperate for the money. By Monday I felt so worried, I hadn't slept, didn't want to eat, and couldn't entertain working with so much on my mind. How could I work being nice to people, acting as if I was OK, when in my mind I was going crazy with worry over how Mike was? Not only that, but I thought that if he needed me it was best I should be here. I could not think of anything worse for him right now, but to try and ring me, and find I couldn't answer the phone; or send me an email and I didn't reply, as I wasn't by my computer. I thought he might only have a few minutes like the other night to contact me, and I wanted to be here for him if and when it happened.

I still had no news on Tuesday, nothing at all. Colin drove round to his house early that morning to see if Mike's car was there, and it was. We even wondered if she had locked him in somewhere so he couldn't contact me. Nothing made sense, all the cars were there. It was so hard for me not knowing what he was going through. Colin and I just kept talking and going over everything. Both of us were confused as to why he wasn't letting us know somehow. The ten o'clock texts had vanished, all communication seemed to have disappeared overnight.

On the Wednesday Colin rang Mike's work; he was told Mike was there, but in a meeting. So we had an idea. If we went over to his work at about 4.30 we could see him when he came out at 5 pm. This way it wouldn't get him into any trouble at home either.

We pulled into the car park of his work and waited. His car was there. Five o'clock created a lot of movement with lots of people leaving. I kept looking up at the windows and doors, waiting for a glimpse of Mike's smiley little face to come running down those steps. I thought he must be so full of things to tell me, either good or bad. I had resigned myself to it probably being bad. I didn't expect anything at this point, I just wanted to know he was safe and well. I also wanted to know what she did or didn't know about me, and whether or not we had any future. I just needed some answers to my questions, that was all.

It was getting later and later and only a few people were left in the building now, and just a few cars left in the car park, including Mike's. It was getting cold and dark. We waited and eventually the last light went out just before about 7 pm. Mike was nowhere to be seen. All the lights were out, and just an empty car left as a reminder of him. We left the premises even more confused than we had been before. I still had not been able to sleep. My mind kept going over everything. The only thing I suppose I was sure of was that he must be OK, as he had driven to work that Wednesday. How he got home was a mystery though.

I couldn't do very much for the next day or so, just the usual waiting for an email or text. The other thing I couldn't understand was that I had emailed him at work, just begging him to write back and let me know he was alright, but he hadn't even replied. I thought if he was worried about her finding out, she wouldn't if it had come from his work email. There was just nothing at all.

Thursday was the same. On the Friday I had to ring the bank to make sure everything was OK with Mike's cheque. I had put it in on the Monday. The bank had the most terrible news. Mike had cancelled it.

I was in a terrible state and everything was now becoming clearer to me. He had not contacted me because he didn't want to. He had cancelled the cheque on me and dropped me right in it. Not only for the £500 he was going to lend me, but also the £100 I had given him to help him that Friday evening so he didn't have to go to the cash point. I started crying on the phone when the bank informed me that it had been cancelled. I was in pieces now, not only over Mike, but also over the money. Bigger worries than before, because this week I had not worked, as I couldn't cope with all the stress.

I became really angry with him for doing that to me as I

thought he loved and cared for me. I understood what he was going through, and would have supported his decision whatever it was, if only he had just told me, instead of breaking my heart. How could he do this to me, when I had got so close? I had let him into my heart, into my world and now he hated me so much he couldn't even tell me what was happening. To top it all, he had dropped me in it big time with the bank, even though half the reason I was so short was because of him.

Just as I finished on the phone with the bank, my dad rang me. I was crying my heart out. He said that Mum and he would help with the money. They were so angry with Mike for dropping me in it. I am not sure what I would have done without their help that day. The bank was really sorry about what had happened. I later went down to see if they could help in any way. However they said that they couldn't at that time. This was one horrible week and I wasn't sure what I had done to deserve it.

The next week was hard. My emotions were going up and down all the time. One minute I really missed Mike and the next I felt angry for what he had done to me. Colin was very good and he tried so hard to be there for me. Sometimes I even pretended to him I was OK. I did a lot of talking, we both did. One night Colin came into the bedroom and found me in bed crying over Mike. I had to work because that was my main priority. I was desperate for the money, more than before. I didn't have any will power; I just wanted to stay in bed thinking, wondering why, and feeling sorry for myself.

However I did manage to work, I tried to just select the nicest customers, the ones that would ask me the least questions and be the least demanding of my time. I didn't feel I had anything to give to people. All the past few years of bad things that had happened to me came flooding back. Bad things of how a friendship of thirty years had gone wrong for me two years ago, and now she didn't even miss me let alone try to put it right. The same happened with another friend from my days at the hospital. I had always been there for him. When things got bad for him, he could always turn to me. Then one day, I don't know why, he wouldn't answer my text messages or ring me. To this day I have no explanation.

Some of my clients were picking up from me that I wasn't right. I tried so hard but failed miserably. I confided in one or two. One in particular was fuming when I told him what Mike had done regarding the cheque, and that day kindly offered to give me more than the usual amount for his massage. This brought tears to my eyes. It reminded me of Mike's kindness before he deserted me. But then reality hit hard on how he had been so hurtful this last two weeks. I tried to refuse the extra money from this client but he insisted, and so I took it. I accepted and thought, "There are still genuine people out there." I told myself, "I must try to think positive."

I didn't trust people very often. I had let Mike in. I had trusted him with my heart and my world. This was the thanks I had back. I wondered how much he hated me now and if he remembered how I didn't let people into my life as a rule. Some days I just felt confused about the whole thing. I wanted him to know that whatever he had decided to do with his life, I would still be here for him. Even though I should hate him, I didn't. I had an idea. I knew he still belonged to the adult website I was on, I knew this because he had in the past left me some ratings. His user name was still there. If he had left the site it would have told me the member was no longer active. I decided to send him an email through the site. I just put in the subject box: "Please Mike if you are reading this please know that I am not cross with you."

Chapter 33
Making Up

After eighteen days of silence I heard from him on the 10th of November 2005. I was at home waiting for work. If I had a withheld number on my mobile I never usually answered them. However this time I did and I said, "Hello." This quiet little voice answered back, "I thought you didn't answer to withheld numbers?"

"Bloody hell, Mike!" I said. "Where the hell have you been, and why did you withhold the number if you didn't think I would answer? Why are you ringing me?"

He replied, "I just had to hear your voice."

I had so many questions and I didn't know where to start. I also wasn't sure how much time he had to talk. He went on to explain how he had tried to give me up. How his partner had gone crazy when she heard what we had done. He said she had completely transformed, and had turned into a loving woman, offering sex on demand. In fact she acted as if she couldn't get enough. He said he wanted to try and make a go of it, but had missed me so badly. They had apparently been away, just the two of them, on holiday to Lanzarote.

She was ill one day and had to stay in bed. This had left Mike to himself and he said it was hard, as there was internet access in the hotel. He wanted to look at my website and write me email. He was desperate to know how I was. I told him I had been so worried, and that I wanted what was best for both of them. I totally understood him trying to make a go of it and agreed he should. I wished him luck and said it was so nice to hear from him after not knowing anything. Now I could and would have to come to terms with it.

Three days later on the 13th of November 2005 he called me again. This time he was dreadfully upset. He said he wasn't coping. He said she had changed so much but it was too late. He said he could not stop loving me, nor could he get me out of his head 24/7. I felt sorry for him. Well actually I felt sorry for them both. If only this had happened many years ago, it would not have been too late for them. I asked him what he wanted me to do.

He said, "I've got to see you. I know I shouldn't but I have to see you again." I agreed to meet him and a few days later we met in his lunch break, at a pub near his work.

He was so pleased to see me and just hugged me for ages. Then we talked some more and the time went so quickly. One of the things I needed to know was why he never came out of work that night when we were waiting for him. He said he had seen us out of the window, and he was worried in case I was mad with him, so he had rung his partner to come and collect him, slipping out the back door. I was upset to hear that. I said he was so far from the truth on why we were there. I also needed to know why he had cancelled the cheque on me. He explained that she had gone through all his money, every account, and wanted to know where every penny had gone. She found out about him giving it to me and made him cancel the cheque. Again I was upset by him not trying to even warn me. But what was done was done. We didn't have very long before he had to return to work.

When I got home Mike had sent loads of emails just like the old days. Then after work, he would write to me from his private email account, telling me how much he still loved me. How he couldn't just give me up.

At home things for Mike were very complicated. His partner was trying to keep up this new woman image. At the same time she was bombarding him constantly with questions, accusations, and pressurising him to hate me. She just wouldn't stop, and day and night she pressurised him. She would ask him questions about me and then when he answered she would not like what he said. He tried everything to make her stop and they kept falling out. Then she would start off from another angle about me.

She had the strangest ideas. One of them was that I was a witch and that he only liked me because I had put a spell on him. I do not know where the hell she got this idea. Perhaps from one of her friends who had been into witchcraft? This woman had apparently put a spell on a married man she was seeing to try to get him to leave his wife. Obviously it didn't work or she wouldn't be on her own now. They were the ones into all the witchcraft it seemed, not me. She even told Mike I had a shop up the road that was into spells and magic. It was a shop about a mile away and she was convinced it was mine. The endless reel of crap that came out of her mouth just went on and on, all the time about me. Mike, instead of agreeing with her, would fight back as much as he could. But he got so tired of hearing it. She would ask every day if he had made contact with me. This I could understand. He did have to lie to her and say no at the time. I later found out she had been driving past my place several times a day and even one of her friends had been outside at seven in the morning. She was getting worse not better. I think she was frustrated, as she had his body but not his mind.

He was back to leading a double life, only this time she had taken his mobile phones off him, thinking that would stop him ringing me. That didn't work either, as he memorised my number, and would call me from a phone box for about twenty minutes every night on the way home from work. If he was at home alone in the evenings, we had worked out a little signal; he would ring twice and hang up. Then I would ring him back so it didn't show up on his phone bill. I was also going over to see him at his work at lunchtime. We would cuddle in the car, or more, and then at night he would go home to her. This went on for a few more weeks. One Friday he got brave and came to our place to see me. I had to laugh as he looked like Mrs Doubtfire. He wore funny clothes and tried to park a long way up the road, so she would not recognise him if she or her friend were watching.

I was finding it hard having Mike some of the time, and knowing he was going home after. I knew he was sleeping and having sex with her now after all those years of abstinence. I felt a bit like she was a new woman in his life, as the old one that he wasn't allowed to have sex with, or touch lovingly, had gone. He used to reassure me by saying, "I don't love her, I love you." He said that when he sat with her on the settee, she would hold his hand. However, with me he would hold it and rub it lovingly. I tried to understand but still found it hard.

A couple of weeks later I had an overnight booking through the adult website. I couldn't speak or email Mike that night. The next morning he was ringing me at 7 am asking if he could meet me at the hotel. He turned up and said, "Now I know how you must feel. Last night was awful." He didn't sleep, as he kept thinking about me lying in the arms of another man for the whole night. I tried to reassure him as I always did; it was just work, and nothing at all emotional. We had breakfast together and he left me for work.

At home not much had changed for the good. She was coming out with more ridiculous ideas and the latest was that he had been doing all the decorating for us. Obviously she didn't know Mike very well. Somehow that's not his thing.

He did his Mrs Doubtfire thing again the following Friday. This time I didn't make him wear a condom. It was the first time we had done sex without protection. Mike was so pleased and came four times, one after the other. He said it was the most emotional moment he had experienced in such a long time. This was Friday the 9th of December. He left here and went to town. He rang me up again on the way home to thank me. I now felt I had given Mike everything.

The next day was the weekend. Saturday came and went with no emails or calls from Mike. I thought it a bit strange, but then thought maybe he wasn't able to escape. Sunday came and went, again nothing from him, not even a little email. I was getting very worried again by now, as two days just didn't figure. He was always so desperate to ring me at every opportunity.

He had told me a few weeks ago that he had booked a family holiday. He said, "I know you are not going to like this, but when it all came out about us, I was trying to make a go of it with her." He had booked for the whole of his family to go to Jamaica.

I understood, and said to him, "Well, you've already made arrangements so you'll have to go." This holiday happened to be on the 13th of December 2005, just two days after this weekend when I hadn't heard from him.

The next morning was Monday the 12th of December 2005. I switched on my computer, and there was the email, the one I had now been expecting. It said she had found out again about us and was going mental. He said we would have to finish for good this time. Apparently she had opened his bank statement and found he had ordered me a personalised necklace in gold and engraved with my name. He had ordered this for me as a Christmas present. She had also seen he had given me back the £600 again after cancelling the previous cheque. That was it; he had been well and truly caught out. He rang me later that day and we said goodbye to each other. He was upset on the phone. I said I would always be here if he needed me and I told him all he had to do was ring me up. He said he was so sorry but he had one more chance to make a go of it with her.

Chapter 34
More Break Ups

I let him go and he made me promise that when the necklace came I would keep it. I said I would, and he told me he would always love me. He also said that he had posted a Christmas card to me, which again he wanted me to keep. She had also found out about that as she questioned him on every transaction that showed up on his bank statement. Unfortunately he had not used cash at the card shop and therefore he admitted it to her. I wished him all the luck with his holiday, telling him it would be hard for me not having him around, and knowing he was going so far away. I wasn't able to have any contact with him now, so he couldn't even tell me which hotel he was staying at. We said goodbye and I felt so sad.

The next day I kept thinking about him going on his holiday with his family. It was also his birthday whilst he was away. I hoped he was having a nice time, but found it bloody hard back here thinking he was happy on a holiday of a lifetime. I felt glad that he was able to do this for his kids though, as they had seen and heard a lot of shit this last few months, with everything that had been going on. I though they deserved some good things to happen now.

Mike and family came back on the 21st of December. On the 23rd he had his works Christmas party in the afternoon. Colin and I were in town shopping when my phone rang. It was Mike. He said, "I still love you."

I said, "You're not supposed to be ringing me up, Mike, are you?" He agreed but said he couldn't help it. He said the holiday had been a disaster from day one and they were constantly arguing, even at the airport before they set off for the long flight. He said that many evenings and nights they had spent time in their room arguing. He said that although they had been to a paradise island, it had not been a good holiday by any means.

I was so shocked. I wasn't really sure how much more messing around I could take. Twice now I had been messed around and twice he had decided to dump me and try and make a go of it with her. Now what was I supposed to do? Should I just tell him to go and get on with it, or should I still be there for him? He sounded so sad, and dreadfully unhappy. I wanted to be with him, but didn't want all the grief either. I was getting all the blame from her and his kids. They all hated me. I could understand why, but if only they had known how many times I had tried to leave him. I knew it would be difficult having contact with him now as he had broken up from work until the 2nd of January. I said, "Well, I'll still be here for you," and we finished talking after about half an hour.

I just couldn't believe it, after all that, he was still not wanting to give me up. With Christmas just a few days away, I didn't know if I was coming or going. Colin and I had arranged to go and stay with my parents for a few days. I took the laptop so I could try and continue my phone chats. Also so I could check my emails from Mike in case he was able to send me any. She was watching him like a hawk now and not letting him out of her sight. Remember, he still had no mobile phone as she had taken it away from him.

Christmas Day came and Colin and I had a nice family get together with my mum and dad. Boxing Day was the same. We had planned to go home the following day and I was just sitting with my mum in her bedroom talking when my mobile rang.

I didn't recognise the number and thought it might have been Mike ringing me from a phone box. I answered it. There was a woman's voice on the other end saying, "Leave us alone, do you understand?" I didn't understand a thing, who was this and what was she talking about? Here it was, a day or so after Christmas, and I was having a nice time with my family when this happens.

Suddenly I realised who it was. It was Mike's partner. My first reaction was anger. I said, "Fuck off, woman, will you."

She replied with "Just remember you said that to me first." I still had no idea what she was on about. She had hung up on me.

A few seconds later it rang again, this time a faint little voice came on. It was Mike. He said in such a quiet tone that I could barely hear him, "We want you to leave us alone." This time I just hung up.

My mum was looking at me, very confused. "What's the matter?" she said. I made some excuse about it being some woman doing cold selling. I said I was so cross, as it was out of order ringing like that over Christmas. She seemed to accept it. I didn't want to say it was anything to do with Mike, and this time I knew for sure, it was certainly not coming from him. Only a few days before he had given me the nicest Christmas card I had ever had; such lovely meaningful words. Also the gold necklace with my name on it was here now and I was wearing it. Plus I had remembered how twice he had tried to give me up but couldn't. I just wasn't sure what had happened to make her say that. It had been over Christmas so it wasn't likely to have been something through the post. Like a bill with my number on it? I was completely baffled. I couldn't wait to speak to Colin who was in the kitchen with my dad. Luckily we were nearly ready to leave for home anyway. All the way home we kept saying, "Whatever has happened now?"

The next day Mike managed to ring me from a phone box. Apparently she had said that someone had been ringing their landline and hanging up on them. She was telling Mike it was me, but of course I had never done any such thing. Why would I do that? For one I was with my family enjoying Christmas, and the other, I already had Mike. I didn't need to act so childish. Even when I didn't have him, it would not have been something I had ever contemplated. If he didn't love me now, ringing his house would not have changed his mind. It would have done the opposite.

New Year's Eve was difficult. I knew Mike and family were

going over to a neighbour's house for the evening. He had managed to sneak a few little emails over to me. We had a great song we both loved by Billy Fury, it was called "A Thousand Stars". He had sent me that song a long time ago. He said on New Year's Eve, although I can't be with you in person, I will be thinking about you and especially at midnight. He told me look up at the stars, find the biggest one you can and that will be me looking down at you. I did look up at the stars that night and remembered his words. As the clock struck midnight, I thought what would next year bring? I was soon to find out.

Chapter 35
He Leaves His Partner

Just into January and Mike returned to work, which was a relief for both of us as it meant we could now write and talk freely. He said his Christmas had been hell on earth. He didn't think things could get much worse, but they had. He had been ordered to get out of bed and kept awake with her questions. She never listened or believed a thing he said. It was constant arguing.

Not long after returning to work, he was asked to go back over to Amsterdam on a business trip, this time with his boss as well. His partner got to hear and insisted on going too, even though he was not on his own. So Mike, not wanting to make a fuss, said, "OK, you can come." I think she was paranoid I was going to go again. He told me it would be hard to go back to the same place, where we had had such a nice time, and to now be going with her. I didn't like the idea myself, as it held good memories of that special trip we had done together. But there wasn't anything I could say or do, I had to accept it.

I found it very hard when they left, wondering what he was thinking. Imagining them in the same hotel as the one we had stayed in. All sorts went through my head. In the meantime I had lent him an old phone of mine as she had still had his. This did come in handy, as he could still send me text messages. They were going to be there two days this time.

On the second day Mike rang me from the airport, and he was at his wits' end. "What's the matter?" I asked. He said he had had such an awful time. She had gone mad in the hotel room, keeping him up all night and going on and on about me, in fact much worse than before. I told him it had been a mistake to take her, as there were too many memories there. He had always agreed with that, but she had been so insistent. He said he was now at breaking point.

I asked, "What do you mean?"

He said, "I have finally had enough." He couldn't take any more. It was now becoming clear to him she hadn't really changed, and she would never ever shut up about me. She wanted him to hate me. He couldn't and therefore it was impossible for him to even think about staying together any longer. He told her he had had enough and wanted to leave when they got back.

They returned and Mike kept up his attitude of wanting to leave. I was surprised. He told her he was going as soon as he could find somewhere to live. I offered for him to stay here if he wanted to leave sooner, and he said he might well take me up on that. She kept finding reasons to delay him. He had the house in his name and had always paid all the bills, ever since they had been together. This was despite the fact that she already owned a couple of other houses, and ran two businesses. She always kept her finances very tight to her chest, not telling Mike how much money she had or what her income was. She did have another plan for Mike though and that was to make him feel extremely guilty, and to make him hand over most of his wages. She had a list of papers written up for him to sign. One committed him to carry on paying for absolutely everything back at the house. She wanted him to pay the mortgage, the gas, the electric, and every other bill. The papers said that this would continue until 6 months after both the children left university. Mike signed it through guilt, and wanting to do the right thing for his children.

On the 27th of January 2006, Mike left the house and rented a little room a couple of miles up the road. Two of his friends were now getting involved; they knew from Mike all about me, my job and everything. One of them said, "You will have to have your own place, you cannot live with her." I didn't really mind either way what he did, as long as he was happy.

The big day came and Mike moved into his room, costing him yet another £300 a month. His daughter asked if he wanted a hand to move the stuff out. He accepted, and then his son said he would help too. The next thing his partner was up at the room also. This all made it increasingly hard for Mike, as he was already upset. I asked him to give me a ring when he was sorted, and Colin and I went over to see if he was all right. He wasn't. He was crying and in a terrible state. I cuddled him and told him it would be hard, but if this is what he wanted I would help and be there for him. He asked if he could come back to our place.

We took him home and cooked him some tea. We tried to make him feel at home, and that we were there for him as much as possible. One thing Mike was not aware of before he left, was Colin's and my sleeping arrangements. For many years Colin and I had not been able to sleep in the same bed together, in fact not even in the same room. Colin had a problem with his legs twitching when he went to sleep. He didn't have this condition when we first met; it developed over the last ten years. Also he had a terrible problem with loud snoring. It too had become very bad over the last few years. Between the two problems it meant sleeping together all night was impossible and we had both accepted it. It didn't stop us loving each other, but it did mean we led a slightly different life to most couples. Colin had slept in the front room for years, leaving me alone in the double bed. Mike was shocked to hear this and I asked if he wanted to stay over with me. After we both explained to Mike how things had been between Colin and I for the last few years, I think he felt a lot more comfortable about how things were with us.

He did decide to stay that night and he needed to be cuddled so tight. I too wanted to look after him and make sure he was coping. I couldn't think of anything worse than him being alone in that room and going through all this on his own. After all it was because of me he had got into this situation.

At first Mike was a complete emotional wreck. I understood this; I had been there myself when I left Patrick. The problem was that it wasn't just hard for Mike, the fact he had left. On top of that, they were back at the house scheming and trying to trick him. It started on day one. His daughter rang him, asking how he was. He was telling her it was hard, and he was very upset. She said she had a problem at home with the computer, she said the screen had gone all funny. Mike tried to help her over the phone by saying try this and try that. She kept saying it wasn't working. Then she asked if he could come over to look as she urgently had to write an important document for a college assignment.

He said, "Yes, can I come now?"

She replied, "No, not until three o'clock as I have to go out now."

He said, "OK, I'll come over at three."

When he arrived he found he had been set up. His partner was there with a best mate of hers and they had a man with them, who his partner claimed was a psychiatrist. She said she had called him in to assess his mental health, as she still thought I had cast a spell on him or hypnotised him. Mike was therefore cornered. (The computer did have a fault, the interface cable to the monitor had been pulled out, which also made him very suspicious.) Next he found this complete stranger asking him all sorts of personal questions. This was one big set-up. It got a bit embarrassing when she kept going on at Mike in front of this psychiatrist about my legs. She told Mike I didn't have legs, I had stumps. She said this in front of everyone, even his two children. She also said that I had put a spell on him and now he couldn't see the real truth. I think, looking back, it should have been her looking at the real truth.

A few days passed, and Mike would still get upset over things, such as if he received a text message from the kids. He felt as if he had lost everything, and was almost homeless. He missed his house and children but did not want to live with his partner.

I tried so hard to look after him. He stayed here with us, and the room he rented remained empty most of the time. We had got into a routine. When Mike came home from work the bathroom was heated nicely for him ready for his shower. The meal would be cooked and just about ready to be dished up for us all. We had even changed our diet a lot to suit Mike, as there was one thing he was fussy about and that was his food. But I never minded that, as we all have things we don't like to eat. I accepted this without a fuss. I had gone from going to bed at any time of the night to going to bed with Mike at 10 pm. This was because after eighteen years of going to bed on his own, I didn't want that for him again. It was hard for me at first, as there were many nights before Mike moved in that I would be up until the very early hours of the morning doing phone chats, or fiddling around changing my website.

He had made arrangements to see his kids in the week, which in the very early days didn't always go to plan. He would usually go around to his old house on a Thursday to see them. It worked OK unless his ex-partner was at home. If she was it would all end in tears. Mike at first would always get upset when he went back home. The worst was when he had to go back at certain times and discuss particular things with his partner. He would go one step forward and three back. Sometimes he was so down he even had thoughts of suicide. This worried me as it was often when he was driving and alone. I felt helpless.

Luckily work was going well for Mike, and not long after moving in he had another trip to Germany. I did ask if I could go too, but he said no, he couldn't afford it. This did upset me, as I had remembered how much he wanted me to go before. I wasn't sure if living with him was a mistake. There were many times I felt I was being taken for granted and that when he didn't have me he wanted me more. We used to lie in bed talking about the summer. He was dreading it as he had a boat and loved water-skiing. He wasn't sure how it was all going to work out for him as his boat was still back at the house.

One thing Mike was beginning to realise was that if he could avoid seeing his ex-partner, he could just manage to keep himself strong. This worked OK as long as she didn't turn up and wait for him to come out of work, and then start having a go at him about something. She always wanted more money. He refused, saying he couldn't give her any more, or he would have nothing left.

When he went round to the house, she was always leaving him notes, trying to make him feel guilty. She had also contacted every one of his friends and tried to get them involved. Some would ring him up and say she had been onto them, but they didn't want to get involved. Others thought they were in some position to make him see sense. She even pestered his eighty-five year old mother, ringing her constantly, and getting her involved. She mentioned to Mike just before he left her, "If you ever take her up to meet your mother I'll tell her all about what she does." This worked with Mike as he didn't want that. He wanted to keep his mother out of all his problems as much as possible, as he was very worried about the emotional effect it was having on her.

So not wanting to rock the boat I had to be kept away. For the first three weeks his mum spoke to me on the phone and even told me to look after him. Then one night when he rang her, she didn't want to know anything or hear anything about me. But all the time his mum was in constant contact with his ex-partner. She even got to writing him notes every week for a while. His mum would say things like how much they all loved him, and please come to your senses and go home. This did used to hurt me. I felt I was doing everything to look after him, and yet his mum and his kids hated me so much. They had no idea to what extent I cared because no one ever gave me a chance to show it. I wasn't allowed to meet his mum. His kids didn't even want to mention my name to him. His work colleagues didn't even know about me. Well only one and that was the woman he had taken out the time we weren't together. I kept asking him if he had told anyone yet and he said no. I said, "Do you think you should say something in case anything happens to you?" He said he would tell the woman, but because they had history he didn't want to tell her in the office. However I wasn't sure of his reasons, because they had now been finished a long time. But he kept insisting he wanted to tell her properly. He asked if I would rather he took her out in the car or went for a walk. I said I would rather a walk. I felt if he got upset it would be easier and that they couldn't get too close. A car could have led to something that was supposed to be over.

He met her for lunch on the 14th of February 2006. The walk I thought was going to be round the industrial estate where his offices were. I was wrong; they went into a wood. He told me how he got upset and she cuddled him. I had my concerns, but mostly kept them to myself at that time.

By now I had quite a few things bothering me. Was I just a convenience, someone to be there and look after Mike? The other was, where exactly did I fit into his world? His family hated me, and also I thought, "Do I trust him?"

Mike didn't only have his main full time job, but two other little businesses as well. It seemed he didn't have a lot of spare time. If he wasn't busy on one job, the other one would take his time. We had some issues over this and I said it was important we spend as much time together as possible, or it wouldn't work. Everything had changed for me. I was no longer getting the lovely cards and treats I had previously been getting. Mike's attitude was, well you have me here now. Sometimes I felt as if I cared for him more than he cared for me. I was doing more and more for him and I had even got into the routine of shaving him and combing his hair before he went to work. I liked making him look his best when he went to work or to meet his kids. I wanted him just to care as much as he used to.

We had endless talks about this. But the one big problem with Mike was no matter how nicely you tried to tell him you were upset about something, he would always take it right out of proportion and see it as the end of the world. I have never in my life had as much patience for anyone as I had for Mike. He would often sulk or want to run away if I was upset about something. I didn't see all this before he moved in as he was the one that always did the chasing.

My biggest fault is my insecurity, I know. I should be more trusting, but life has made me insecure. If Mike ever did anything like being late home it would start my insecure mind off. I wanted to trust him, but I keep telling him that trust has to be built up over time, it doesn't just happen overnight. I think it would have helped if I had truly felt he loved me and started to show it more. For the last twenty years Mike had been used to doing what he liked whenever he liked, as she didn't care enough to even question where he had been. On the other hand

I am completely the opposite to him. I have said to him, "If I didn't care I wouldn't care where you were either." I found at times he had been so used to doing his own thing, he could at times be very selfish. We did discuss and iron out a lot of these issues, and he did try after he had picked his pride up off the floor, to take on board my concerns and try harder with me.

As well as the bad times we have had some tremendous good times over this last year. We joined a health and fitness club nearby, as one thing Mike was missing when the sun shone was his swimming pool. We joined this club in May and spent hours over the summer around the pool sunbathing and with him being able to go for a swim when it was really hot. I found it a little hard at times as I had a bad foot and wasn't able to entertain going in the water, even when it was boiling hot. I enjoyed watching Mike, he was happy, we were both happy. We had a little secret thing up there where we would talk to each other about the people around the pool. It was so funny, we even gave them false names as we didn't know their real ones. We made a little rule that we would try and avoid speaking to people at the club, so we could go up there and get some peace, as we were limited in where we could just be alone together.

Chapter 36
The Holiday

We spent as much time as we could out in the summer, as it meant we could be alone together. Of course it had the added benefit of letting us enjoy the sunny weather.

Things at home had become a little strained, not on Colin's side so much but on Mike's. He found he wanted to spend more and more time with me alone, and so at every opportunity we would eat out. We found an offer on at the local pub up the road where they did a "two for one" meal, so we took advantage of that most days. It worked out cheaper in a lot of ways than shopping, cooking and eating at home. Colin didn't seem to mind, although looking back I was stuck in the middle, feeling guilty for being out all the time and leaving him on his own so much. It was getting hard as I wasn't sure who I should be keeping happy. The summer meant Mike could also meet up with his children and take them water-skiing some mornings and evenings when the weather was fine.

Mike and I still had our problems, although he had settled down from a lot of the guilt he had previously been experiencing. Sometimes he would like to spend time doing what he wanted rather than compromising and seeing if I was happy. I loved going to the swimming pool and sunbathing, but not every single day. I felt sometimes as if I was afraid to ask to do something else, and if I did he would say he wanted to go to the pool anyway. We did have talks about this, and he did compromise in the end, spending some days doing other things.

When my foot got better I asked Mike if he would try and

teach me to swim. He agreed with enthusiasm. It was also around about July when he came home from work one Friday afternoon excited. He had managed to get hold of some extra money, something to do with him changing the mortgage over from his old house. He said, "Do you fancy going on holiday?"

I was delighted and said, "I'd love to."

We went up to the pool that day really excited about where we were going to go. We were obviously on a budget, but never the less we were still going on holiday. I have always loved going away and it was something to look forward to. At that particular time we seemed so close and happy, and although things were not perfect we were finding ourselves getting on really well.

Not long after this we started to run into difficulties again. I am not sure what created it but we had some issues, and the holiday wasn't brought up by either of us. I didn't push it, as I felt perhaps he had changed his mind, as he didn't mention booking it. One thing with Mike was if he made his mind up about something he would always get on and do it straight away and he rarely put things off. It was a quality I had always liked about him, but on this occasion it irritated me, as I thought he was putting off booking the holiday.

In the end I actually said to him, "Don't worry about the holiday, I don't know if I want to go now." This went on for a few weeks and again he didn't seem to push the issue. Now I was really beginning to think he had changed his mind. In the beginning we had had a quick look on the internet and found some places to go, but he hadn't committed to booking anything, so again I didn't push it.

We were again running into problems and I felt now he didn't want to take me. This had a knock-on effect, as that made me more insecure, causing us to drift apart again. Another month had gone by, and we still hadn't really committed to this bloody holiday. I was always too worried to say anything to him as whenever I did he would always take it the wrong way, and then neither of us would talk about how we felt. Me for fear of upsetting him, and him for being selfish and always feeling sorry for himself instead of thinking about how I felt.

On top of this we still had the other issues of his kids hating me, and he would still have to leave me out of his life regarding anything he had to do with them. His friends at work still didn't know about me, apart from a couple of them. Therefore I still felt very excluded and isolated, whereas it wasn't like that for him. All my family, my children and my parents knew Mike and seemed to accept and like him. Although nobody at this point had asked questions, it was becoming more obvious to everyone that we were together all of the time.

A few more weeks went by and eventually I mentioned the holiday. He then agreed to book it but did ask me, "If I book it and we do split up, do you promise you would still come as I don't want to waste the money?"

I said, "Of course I would."

So we picked a holiday to Gran Canaria off the internet, going out at the end of September. I felt relieved that he had finally done it as it showed me he had committed to me a little.

Now it was time for me to start the swimming. So about a week before we went, my foot was better enough for me to go into the water. After spending a boiling hot summer around the pool, just watching and overheating, I was now finally going to be able to get in and see how I got on.

We both agreed I should go in the indoor pool and at a quiet time, so we ended up going in the evening. This was the first time I had been in a swimming pool for many years. I was clinging onto Mike for dear life. Eventually I got a bit braver and tried to see how I felt going right under the water. I had never been right under before so this was a new experience for me. I managed it, and Mike was really pleased with me. I went a few more times before the holiday, but never achieved the confidence to let go of him.

It was now time for the holiday and we were so excited, all packed and ready to go. We went up to Gatwick and stayed the night before so as not to make the day of flying too stressful. Everything went to plan and next we were on the plane taking off to the lovely island.

The flight went really well. I was so excited, we both were, and it was also a chance for us to have a complete week alone, away from everyone. The hotel was fantastic, all inclusive, and the weather was glorious. In fact when we arrived that evening, we thought the air conditioning wasn't working, but it turned out they had had a heat wave, sending it up well over a hundred degrees.

Each morning we went down to the pool after breakfast, and found a spot suitable for me, as I needed to be as close to the pool as possible. Although Mike had to help me, we found a way for me to get into the pool. I would sit on one of the mattresses they used on the sun beds and he would drag that with me on top over to the pool. I was then able to climb in. We had bought a large rubber ring so I could be independent whilst in the pool. It was great, although I must have looked so funny bobbing about. I would be in there for an hour and a half on my own sometimes, and once I got in I didn't want to get out.

One day they were doing water aerobics and I had an idea that if I got in the middle of them all, maybe I could join in. This went terribly wrong and before I knew it, I was kind of trapped in the middle of them all and thinking, "Shit, now how am I going to get out of this one?" The trouble was that in the ring I could only paddle backwards, so I could never see where I was going and kept bumping into people. Eventually I did escape from the aerobics class while Mike was laughing his head off at me. I think I was laughing too, as how could I ever have thought I could do water aerobics without the use of my legs? I think when I was in the water surrounded by all those people, I felt equal, because for once in my life I was seeing everybody at eye level. This was a new experience and one I hadn't been used to. Only when it came down to it, I soon found I still couldn't use my legs as they could. Strange how the water made you forget.

Our week continued to go well, and we made a few friends along the way. They would watch us around the pool as Mike helped me, cheering us on and helping if we needed it. This week was a real test for Mike and me, as it was the first time he had been responsible for me without the help of Colin. We managed fairly well although there were times I missed Colin, as although Mike is good he isn't quite as understanding and caring as Colin. Perhaps it was the lack of being used to dealing with a disabled person; after all Colin had been around me for seventeen years.

Coming home, I think Mike found it even harder; after having me to himself for a week, he now had to go back to sharing me again. He was thinking about my job and knowing we were going home to a shared house. When we were home we had now started to spend a lot of the time in the bedroom alone. We had a TV in there, so after eating out, we would come home and just retreat to the bedroom. This way I felt Mike could cope with Colin being around. I felt totally helpless and in the middle, not knowing who I should be keeping happy. I didn't want to upset or hurt anyone's feelings, I just wanted everyone to be happy, but I suppose this was just not going to happen.

Chapter 37
Attempted Suicide

The next few months went by and things were worse after the holiday than before. On returning from holiday and having Mike to myself, I found that he was snowed under with work. Mike had a business on the side apart from his main job and a particular problem had come up that needed his immediate attention. He had to travel to Birmingham the next day and was not sure if he would be back that night. I felt a bit frustrated as I understood he had to work and his full time job required him to be away for nearly eleven hours a day. Now the other one was taking up a lot of time also, and still there were his children to fit in. Therefore I was feeling rather low about it all. This caused us to fall out and he could never understand why I felt like I did. I would explain over and over, if this is going to work between us I need to have quality time. But he was not convinced and carried on doing what he had to do.

In the November things came to a big head. I was feeling insecure and not sure how much he really wanted me in his life. We fell out one day, leading to him saying the words I had been waiting for: "I want to leave." I wasn't shocked as deep down I had always felt it was just a matter of time. He explained that he didn't really know how he felt and I think the mistake had been that he hadn't had any time on his own after he first left his family. I don't think he really knew for sure at this point if he could manage to live on his own, and not have me in his life. Mike often wanted the good times without the bad, and without me asking any questions or not having my say, if I didn't like something or felt unhappy about a situation. I had found out he had lied to me on one occasion about an email he had received at work from an old friend. When I questioned him about it he didn't like it. This led to an argument and so he decided he didn't want the grief and said that he wanted to leave me. He packed his things up and left that Friday afternoon. I felt awful as he left, I was crying but it didn't make any difference, he still wanted to go.

That night he texted me and said he had rented a room and he missed me, but didn't say he wanted to come back. On the Saturday we spoke on the phone, and I said I would give him two weeks to make up his mind about how he felt about me, and if he wanted to come back he could. He was grateful and came around to pick up the rest of his things. We talked and cuddled as he left. I felt so empty, as one minute he was there in my life the next he wasn't. I looked around our room and it felt empty with all his things missing. I told myself I had to be strong and carried on the rest of the day hoping he still loved me. That night he texted me: "I am coping, because I know you are still there in my life."

On the Sunday morning, I woke up feeling really odd, I cannot explain how I felt, just not right. I rang Mike to see how he was coping and he sounded fine on the phone. He said he had slept well and felt OK and I said I was glad. I didn't stay on the phone long as I wasn't coping and I didn't want him to know. I said, "Goodbye, Mike," and hung up.

My heart was racing and my head was spinning, I didn't know what to do. The only thing I wished for was that I wasn't in this world any more, hurting people and causing people so much anguish and sorrow.

Without another thought I grabbed all the sleeping tablets I could find, and counted them out onto the bed. I grabbed a glass of water and took three there and then. Then I started to count the amatriptyline tablets I had been prescribed from the doctor for my migraines, and made a huge pile on the bed. I decided now to have a very quick shower as fast as I could. As I ran the water over me, the only thought I had in my head was, "I want to get the hell out of this world." I didn't even consider or think about anyone else.

The three sleeping tablets I had already taken had started to kick in and I went from my heart racing frantically to feeling very calm and almost at peace. Just then my mobile rang, it was Colin, and he was ringing to see how I was. He was at the market and had a quiet patch and wanted to see if I was OK. I tried to act normal, but he said, "You sound all slurry, are you OK?" I said I was fine and tried to act normal.

When I hung up, I turned my phone off. I then started to take the rest of the tablets, shovelling a handful down at a time. I knew I had about seven hours before anyone would find me. The only thing I hadn't done was write a note to everyone to say I was sorry. I found a pad and paper, but I was starting to lose the plot. Writing quickly, I wrote one to Colin telling him how sorry I was to do this to him. One to Mike to say that now I was out of his life forever he could be happy, and the last to my son and daughter telling them I loved them and how sorry I was to do this to them and begging them to forgive me.

After that I vaguely remember trying to get dressed. I can just recall hearing Mike's voice and then felt an almighty smack to my face. I don't recall another thing after that until later that evening, when a nurse was leaning over my bed calling my name and asking if I knew where I was. I was so angry, thinking, "What the fucking hell am I doing here?" This was not supposed to have happened. I didn't want to be here. How had I got to the hospital?

Apparently the alarm bells had started to ring when Colin called me from the market. He wasn't convinced that I was alright, and as hard as I had tried to sound normal on the phone, I hadn't pulled it off. He had tried to call me back and found the phone switched off. He then called Mike and said can you go round there quick as I don't think she is OK. Mike had got here first but couldn't get in as I had left the key in the door to stop anyone from entering. Mike was at the back door, trying to take the hinges off, when Colin arrived. When they finally got in I was found unconscious on the floor in the living room. I must have heard Mike calling me and tried to get up. I had then fallen to the floor which is how I remember hurting my face. Somehow I had crawled into the front room before I finally went completely unconscious. In the process I had badly grazed and cut my lip and legs and had blood running down my face. Colin and Mike called 999 and an ambulance came. I don't know what they did to me in the ambulance, but they worked on me for about twenty minutes outside the house before taking me to the emergency room at the hospital.

The next day was very much a blur, as I had discharged myself from the hospital against their advice. I don't remember going home, or being put to bed that night, although I remember Mike sat on my bed at home sometime that night, telling me he was going to move back in. I spent the whole of the next day sleeping, just aware that Colin was in the room. Mike rang me in his lunch break to see how I was, and apparently I was very down, but again I don't remember the conversation with him.

By the evening I had started to come round more. Colin said the hospital were worried about me, and had rung to see how I was. Mike gave up the room he had taken on the Friday and said he was sorry for hurting me, and he wanted to come back.

I know how I have felt down in the past over different things that have happened to me, and like everyone I had felt low at times. However never before had I felt so frustrated, hurt and confused at what everyone expected from me.

A couple of days later I was alone on a bus, looking around and thinking to myself, "Why am I still here?" and I wondered what my future would be. I kept thinking, "There must be a reason why I was saved that day." I was still asking myself lots of questions about Mike: why he had returned to me, was it because he felt he had to, or was he genuine in that he did want to be with me? He did at the time seem genuine, and so I slowly started to feel myself again.

The doctor had asked to see me, to talk through why I did what I did, and I explained the whole truth to him. He was surprised I had sunk so low, as I had always been so level-headed before, but on reflection, the doctor seemed to totally understand, and said if I needed to talk further he would be there.

Chapter 38

Playing Away

It was coming up to Mike's birthday in December, and this would have been the first time I would be able to celebrate it with him. I had wanted to do lots of things for his special day, firstly because it was the first time I had been able to, and also because when he was with his partner she would always make him promises and never carry them through.

At one time he mentioned having a helicopter ride, or a flying lesson. I had been looking on the internet for a long time, but he kept saying, "No, it's too much money for you and I don't need it." I felt sad that he didn't want me to treat him, but at the time with my money worries he was right to have persuaded me not to spend out even more. He was grateful to me for just buying him a nice meaningful card.

On the day of his birthday his children were away on holiday, but had left him cards and presents to open. I wanted to get up and make him a special cooked breakfast. We were always alone in the house on a weekend as Colin was at the market and luckily his birthday had fallen on the Sunday. Mike opened his cards from his family, and became very upset, making him reflect over what had happened. He felt sad that they could not be with him, and also sad as the year before they had all been on holiday together. I understood how he felt and tried to comfort him. But instead of giving him a really good and happy birthday it ended up making both of us feel really sad.

The next big event for us was Christmas. How were we going to handle this one? My parents saved the day a little, as we were invited over to their house for the day. It was easier than Mike, Colin and I being at home for the day, as I knew Mike wouldn't have felt comfortable with this. It also meant he was off work for a couple of weeks for the Christmas holiday. I was worried about this too as I knew he had let a lot of his holiday from work go, rather than taking it to be left at home with Colin and myself.

We managed to get through it, and the time went by fairly quickly. He took the opportunity to visit his mum, and although I wasn't allowed to visit her with him, I did go to her home town with him and stay in a hotel. Whilst he spent a few hours with her, I would often change my website address to specify the town where I was now staying. It was quite convenient to be able to do this, as it stopped me from being bored and also helped pay towards the room. On this occasion the phone was going mad. I often went away making this arrangement, and when I got there I would change my mind or lose my bottle. On this occasion Mike left me at about midday, and I had taken a few calls, but I didn't like the sound of them. I was not sure if I would be safe and so I made an excuse that I was busy. Then I had a call from another man, he sounded nice, not too pushy, I asked if he would call back at three thirty as I needed some time to get my head around whether I really wanted to do this kind of thing today.

Some days I would wake up and feel I looked like shit, and my confidence would be very low about myself. This was one of those days. I looked in the mirror of the hotel, and thought, "Who would want to pay money for having sex with me today?" It was the sort of day when everything felt wrong. I was feeling fat, my hair didn't look right, and my makeup didn't seem to be perfect. So eventually I would talk myself out of it. It got to three-twenty; I hadn't eaten, and I had now made up my mind not to go through with this booking. I went over to the restaurant and ordered a meal; with my mobile in my hand I decided I would send him a very kind text explaining that I was very sorry, but I was unable to make the appointment.

No sooner had I sent the text to him when he rang me back. "Oooops," I thought, "now I'm going to have to explain properly."

After saying I was not able to see him, I felt really guilty, as he explained he was only five minutes away. I then went on to say I wasn't feeling as good as I should, and I only like to see men when I look my best.

He said, "Look, I'm not bothered about that." He went on to tell me how nice I sounded on the phone. He knew I was in a wheelchair, and nothing was going to put him off.

In the end I said, "Look, just give me twenty minutes, and I'll see you." I gulped my dinner down and went back to my room as fast as I could, trying to clean my teeth, brush my hair and put the rest of my sexy underwear on.

A few minutes later he rang to find out which room I was in. I was lying on the bed waiting for him. In walked one of the most handsome men I have seen as an escort. He was tall, dark and just lovely. "Wow, this has got to be a perk of the job," I thought, "there aren't many, and he's just so good looking that I can't understand why he needs to pay for sex." I introduced myself and took the money, and then turning my attention to him I slowly undressed him. I was still thinking, "Oh my god, I must have died and gone to heaven." He said he loved my pictures, especially my eyes and that was what had drawn him to my profile. This comment wasn't new to me, as most of the men I saw told me it had been my eyes that drew them to me.

He then started stroking my breast and rubbing his hand up my leg. By the bulge in his trousers I could see how turned on he was. "What do you like best of all?" I asked, groaning.

He replied, "Suck my cock, please," and so without hesitation I knelt down in between his legs. I took his hard throbbing tool into my hand and slowly lowered my red lips over it, gently sucking and going deeper and deeper down into my throat. I could feel he was close to coming, and not wanting to make it happen before his time was up, I slowed right down. I just teased the end of his cock with my tongue while looking up at his handsome face. I started to smile and get on top of him, rubbing my now exposed tits over his cock and chest on the way up until I reached his face. Then I shoved my hanging breasts into his mouth and asked him to suck them while looking down at his gorgeous face, as he took my tits into his mouth. I was on the point of bursting myself. I then slid his cock into my very wet pussy and told him to fuck me harder and harder. We both came at the same time, nearly screaming the hotel down. We were both exhausted for a few moments afterwards and needed to get our breath back.

He started to get dressed and as he did, we began to talk. I asked him why a man as handsome as himself would need to pay for sex. He told me he was never very confident at chatting women up, and that it was easier for him to just pay for it. He then went on to tell me, how he had become addicted to seeing prostitutes. He said that over the last twenty years he had become so hooked on it he couldn't stop. I asked if he had a girlfriend and if so, would that make him stop? He then surprised me by saying that he did stop for a year, but then sadly went back to it. In fact he told me that now it was worse than before, leading to the breakdown of his relationship with his girlfriend. He seemed very down about the whole thing and told me that after the New Year, he was going to try desperately hard to stop seeing prostitutes. He even said he was going to try to do something with the computer so he wasn't able to access the sites as this was the root of the problem. He went on to tell me that he would start by just looking at the girls' profiles on the computer, and then before he knew it, he was so driven by something inside him, that he felt compelled to go out and book one.

This story was one I had heard from many men, and they all said the same. How they had tried it and before long they were addicted to seeing more and more women. Most of them were happily married and even told me how much they loved their wife and kids, but they just couldn't help themselves. This used to worry me a lot, as hearing all these different tales from so many different men made me wonder if Mike might have felt like this at times too. Having experienced seeing prostitutes before, he used to joke with me and say, "I live with one now, don't I? I don't need to pay for it any more." Although Mike desperately wanted me to give up escorting, so that he didn't have to share me any more. There was another part of him, however, that I felt would think I wasn't so exciting if all the naughtiness had disappeared.

Long after the appointment time was over, I was still happy to talk to this client about his feelings. I felt I wanted to help him, but being so far away from my home town I wasn't sure how. He left about an hour and a half later and I wished him good luck as he went out the door.

Chapter 39
Money Worries

Mike returned from his mum's after having had a nice day with her. We talked about my client and how he had problems with his addiction to prostitutes. He said he could understand that feeling, and hoped he would never again be in the position of wanting to visit one. He reassured me that he wanted to put his past behind him. We had a nice evening together and took our time driving back the next day.

Money was playing a huge part on my mind now as my mounting debts were getting harder to deal with. Sometimes I would try to put the worries to the back of my mind. I was always extremely organised, and although it was hard, I always did manage to pay my debts on time. However I was only able to make the minimum payments, but it meant everyone was happy and not aware how difficult it was for me.

One day Mike and I sat down and worked out how much I owed. This was something I hadn't actually done before. I knew it was probably a lot but I was totally unaware of the exact amount. We were both shocked. I was crying and said, "I don't know what to do." It was clear I would never be able to pay them off. Even if Mike did want to commit to me, with all that debt around my neck, it was impossible to expect him to deal with this. It was getting critical, as I was already working as much as I could manage, doing both the escorting and the massage. It was harder for me now as Mike lived with me as well, which meant my hours were more restricted than before. He worked in the day, but before I would work more in the evenings as well as the day, so I found I was doing fewer hours and needed more money. Also I had virtually given up doing the phone chats as again my time was limited, I didn't like to do them when anyone was around, as I found this distracting, and I wanted to give the men that booked me the best. This did involve a lot of concentration and peace and quiet to be able to concentrate on the scenario they requested.

Each month the bills were coming in and each month I was scraping the barrel to make the minimum payment. Often I would lay awake at night worrying, but I didn't say anything to Mike as I didn't want him to worry and feel he was at all responsible. By now it was fundamentally impossible to continue to meet my rising debts. I put on a brave face to everyone, but inside I was beside myself with the stress and worry of it all. Some days the phone didn't ring at all and I would get up and get ready, and then just sit there and wait. I would lose the will to live, let alone work. By the time it got to about three o'clock in the afternoon, and knowing Mike would be home in just two and a half hours, I would be really depressed, knowing that I hadn't taken a penny. Then the next day I would get loads of calls which would make up for the day before. At that point I would breathe a sigh of relief and wonder why I had worried so much the day before.

I would often get an offer of a loan through the post or an increase to my credit cards. This would be great news as it meant I could use the money not to enjoy myself with, but to help pay the bills that month, taking some of the pressure off working. I knew the following repayments would be hard but at the time I thought I would do it for now and worry about the statements when they came in. In the meantime, I was hoping for some miracle. "Maybe I'll win the lottery," I thought and then my money worries would be over.

January also brought some more strains upon Mike and me. Stupid things, like he had started to leave earlier in the morning than usual. I took it the wrong way partly because of my lack of trust, as when I think back that was what he used to do to his ex-partner when he was seeing me. I still had to remember what he was capable of, with all the lies and deceit that had happened before. He always reassured me he would not do that to me, but I found it hard to believe as trust has to be built up with me over a long period of time. This was partly due to the things that had happened to me when I was a child. The first morning I said, "Why are you leaving this early as you don't have to be there until eight?" and he answered, "Because the traffic is getting bad."

This continued all week, which really bugged me, as he had been with me months and only now had he changed his routine. He got angry when I mentioned it and said he did not like not being trusted. I tried to explain that it was because I cared that I questioned him, and I said, "If I didn't care, I'd just let you get on with it and never say a word, just like it was with your ex-partner."

After a few days of dwelling on it, I remembered that he had previously seen a woman at work, although admittedly it was when we weren't together. Therefore I wasn't completely satisfied with his reasons. I asked myself, was it so he that he could go and check his personal email account before he started work, as maybe he didn't want to do it in front of me? We had had some issues previously about this too. He used to write to me from a secret email account. One day when I asked him what he used it for now, he said "Nothing." I later found out he had been on some adult dating sites, and occasionally still received emails into that account. He said the reason that he didn't tell me was because he had received emails from previous women, although not for a long time, and he was still worried that one might still try and contact him again. Every time I found something out I would ask him to tell me if there was anything else I should know about or any other sites. He would say no, nothing, and then a few months later I would find yet another one. He would say he had forgotten about it and get all upset and angry. This of course didn't help me and my suspicious mind.

After the first four days of him leaving early, I decided to leave the house just after him, not to follow his car but to see how bad the traffic was. I wanted him to be right. I wanted to be stuck in traffic. But each morning it didn't matter what time I left, it took about eighteen to twenty minutes to get to his work. I didn't say anything for a while between the arguments about whether or not he wanted me to care or not.

I decided that for a couple of weeks I would show him how it would be if I didn't care. For the first few days I asked him nothing at all, I didn't say I loved him and I didn't show him that I was interested in what he looked like. I even left him to shave himself, as this was something that I used to do for him every morning. By the end of two weeks we had become very distant and ended up not knowing what to say to each other. He had stopped asking me what my day had been like and I did the same. We were like two strangers, he had his thoughts and I had mine.

One Friday evening we had gone up to the pub for our usual "two for one" dinner and he asked me how long I was going to keep up this "I don't care" attitude. I still had it on my mind about the time it took him to get to work, and so I asked him again why he left earlier and again he gave me the same story as before. I then told him what I had done, taking the same journey at approximately the same time. He went absolutely mad and said, "I can't live like this anymore, I want to leave you." I asked if it was because I had found out how long it does take him, and he just kept saying, "I am leaving and I have had enough." I then gave him a piece of my mind, telling him that he wanted it all his own way, he was selfish, and if that was what he wanted then he could go and get on with it.

We talked for a couple of hours and both calmed down but he was still insisting that he was leaving me. Even sitting outside the house at eleven o'clock that night, I said, "Is there any way you're going to change your mind, and we can sort this out?"

He said, "NO."

I asked what he wanted to do then, and he said he would collect some things and leave now. I said, "Well if that's the case you can take the bloody lot," as I didn't want him to come back the next day like the last time and collect the rest of his stuff.

We both went in and I was so mad with him. I threw most of his things on the bed, saying "Fucking leave then." I had never reacted like this to him before. I asked him to put his computer on, and I then deleted as many of my pictures as I could find. I said to him if you don't want me then you will not want to be looking at these either. He left with his car full of stuff at about 1 am. This time I wasn't upset, I was livid. I was so angry this time and I was determined to let him go for good.

The next day, which was a Saturday, I made no contact and neither did he. I decided to join some dating agencies. There was one that I had already joined before, not to find anyone, but it was to do with looking up a friend we both knew was on there. So I reactivated this site and updated my details. I set about writing to as many men as possible and I couldn't believe the response. I received over five hundred emails in a few days, all saying they would take me out on a date. "Maybe it's time I had some fun," I thought, "after the year I've just had."

I had arranged a couple of dates with some men I liked the sound of. Colin didn't mind as we had become like brother and sister by now, and having gone through this with Mike he just wanted me to be happy. On the Sunday I had arranged to go to the market with Colin, and he was going to pick me up at eleven. When he collected me he said, "You're not going to like what I have to tell you."

"What is it?" I replied.

He said Mike had been up to the market to see him and to drop off a couple of my items he had found in his things. Colin then went on to say, "You'll never guess where he's living?"

I had no idea, and a few things ran past my mind, perhaps he was back at his old room he had rented when he first left? In those few seconds I couldn't understand the anger in Colin's voice. With that I said, "I don't know. I can't imagine, tell me."

"He's only gone back home," he replied, "back to his ex-partner's house."

I just sat there totally stunned. So stunned I was speechless. Suddenly I panicked as I realised I was on my way up to a public place where I couldn't cry and I had to put on a brave face. I couldn't think of anything worse at that moment in time. "I can't do this," I said to Colin.

He totally understood and said, "I'm so sorry, I don't know what to do as I can't leave the market, but also I don't want to leave you at home alone."

I decided that as we were nearly there I would get out of the car, but not go in the market. I told Colin I was just going to wander around by myself, just alone for a while, to gather my thoughts. After he left this time, I wasn't going to ring Mike. I had been a lot stronger, but hearing this news made me so mad that I rang his mobile. There was no answer so I left a voice message telling him I thought he had hated me but now I was convinced he did. I also sent him a text message saying the same.

About half an hour later, I was wandering around the houses near the market and still not wanting to face people. My mobile rang. It was Mike. He said, "I don't hate you, far from it."

He explained that when he left me that night he had driven to a car park, and then he had driven past his ex-partner's new boyfriend's house to find her car was outside very early in the morning. So then he texted his son, asking him if they could meet up. When they got together, they talked about him going back to live there. Basically he thought the situation was now very different, since his ex-partner now had a new man in her life and spent many nights round at his place. Therefore his son and daughter were mostly left at the house on their own. He thought that now his ex-partner would no longer care what he did and might not object to this arrangement; after all it would ensure that he kept paying the bills. He discussed this arrangement with all three members of his family and they all initially agreed. When he explained all this to me I did understand, and could understand how it had happened even if I didn't like it.

We spoke on the phone for half an hour, and then he came up to the market to meet me. He said he still loved me and that he didn't know how it was going to work out with him living back at the house. He was sleeping in the spare room, his ex-partner at first didn't seem too bad, but within a day started to give him a hard time. It was also quite clear she still hated me, in fact more so than she had before. The following day she was screaming in his face, "You're a fucking liar!" and told him she wanted him to leave. His son said at that point that if he went then he would go with him, and with that she calmed down.

He stayed a few more days and during one of them he took me out swimming. I had told him I had gone onto the dating sites, and was going to go out on some dates as we were over, he had finished with me. He accepted this and in the evening would write to me or text me from his room. He had confided in his son everything about me. They had a lot of heart-to-heart talks and they got much closer.

His son said he would go and live with him, as it was clear that Mike couldn't carry on living there. Mike was in contact with me, and his ex-partner knew this as he wasn't lying anymore. She twisted the situation and said he had only gone back there to try and get the house, and that we had both planned it. She of course was so wrong. On the Friday Mike packed up all his belongings from their house and went to work. He texted and rang his son, asking him to contact him as soon as possible so he could decide if he was going to look for a place for both of them to live. Unfortunately he heard nothing back.

I asked him to ring me when he left work, and when he called I asked, "Where are you going to go?" He said that he didn't know, and I asked if he would like to come back to me until he heard from his son. He said that it didn't seem fair as it appeared he would be using me. I said, "Well, that's the risk I'm going to take, as I don't want you on your own, lonely in a bed and breakfast somewhere, or feeling as if you have nowhere in the world to go."

He came back and it was just as well as he didn't hear from his daughter until the Sunday, and nothing from his son until the following Thursday. At this point he still didn't know if his son wanted to live with him. Mike and I had talked, and he explained that he was at the point now where he wanted a place of his own. With all this turmoil we had again got close. He was now in a quandary, because he had committed to living with his son, but wanted us to move in together as a proper couple. I agreed that if his son didn't feel he could still leave and live with him, then I would accept and go with him.

That week was very hard as none of us knew what was happening. He met up with his son on the Thursday. His son was in a real state, he was feeling torn as his mother was making him feel very guilty, and reminding him how much money she was spending on him each month. The crunch day came when he met his son and talked it through. Although his son had made a promise, he didn't feel he could go through with it, and all the consequences that would follow.

At last now we knew where we all were. Mike and I set about looking for a suitable place for him to live. One thing that had changed was his commitment to his house. Since he left he had been paying every single bill including the cable TV with all the options. His ex-partner had been pleading poverty and this had made him feel very guilty. However he found that she had invested a large sum of money in her new boyfriend's property and this made him feel very angry and used. He therefore decided to stop paying all the bills except for the mortgage and house insurance. This of course freed up a lot of money that would now allow him to rent a one bedroom flat or bungalow.

I still had a lot of negative thoughts at times, and one was, "Did he choose me because his son changed his mind?" I have to live with that thought to this day. "Was I second best?" Plus when I had first gone out with Patrick and he got his first flat, he didn't want me around, so all those memories came flooding back.

Eventually he found a little bungalow not too far from my place with Colin. We got the key and Mike included me fully in the setting up of the place, even buying a bed that was suitable for me with my disability. He also made some ramps to make the access to the front door easier. Colin was initially upset and very worried that he wouldn't see me. I kept reassuring him that he would see me every day as I still had to go home and work, as both Mike and I agreed that I would not work from his place. This all went to plan and Colin could see I was still around every weekday.

I have found it difficult at times, sometimes wondering where I really live as I have things at both bungalows. My debts were still hanging around my neck and now living in two places made it even harder to meet the demands. I had started to write this book on the 31st of December 2006, hoping I could find a way of making enough money to pay off my debts before I sunk. However sadly it was impossible and on the 10th of April 2007, I was no longer able to cope and declared myself bankrupt.

Looking back over my life, I have been taught many things. Some have been huge mistakes I have made, in the way I have dealt with events, especially where my emotions are concerned. Other mistakes have been in the way I have handled money, feeling at times money could buy happiness. All these things have taught me to take a good look at myself, and reflect on how I have coped with issues close to my heart. I want to try and learn from my mistakes and use these past experiences to make me a better person. It's funny the things that get you down, my wheelchair never bothers me now. However I must admit to sometimes getting a little depressed about some of my other problems, such as constant headaches and problems caused by very bad circulation.

Over the last few months many more dramatic events have happened, some for the good and some for the bad. For those of you reading this book that know me personally, you will realise how sad I feel at times over the hurt that has been caused to me and also the hurt I may have caused to them. One thing I have learnt is that we cannot go back – we can only ever move forward and try to forgive, and maybe find a little space in our hearts to remember we have all at some time in our life hurt someone.

Reflecting back over these past events in my life, I feel that it has made me a much stronger person. Regrets are only there if it has involved someone else, maybe I have hurt others at times and for those times I would like to say sorry and I wish I could change the way things happened.

I have no regrets for the way life has been to me, for the suffering as a child, the growing up and finding my way in this world. I feel it has moulded me to have empathy towards those that suffer physically in life. It has made me a caring person who can relate to most circumstances. Also I try not to be too judgmental of others, as I know I too have gone down a path that some would regard as bad. I do not have too many regrets on this, as I was as the book is called: *Born Naughty*. There were times I feel I was putting my life on the line, regarding safety, and sometimes when I didn't feel good about myself, and wished I didn't have to do this for money.

Because of my decision to declare myself bankrupt I no longer have to work as an escort to meet my mounting debts. This has been a huge relief to me and all my family who now know the job I was doing in secret for two years. I thank them for the support they have shown me and not judging me too harshly.

I still do the massaging which does gives me a sense of achievement, as I am greatly appreciated by a large number of people. If this book was to be successful, however, it would be so nice to not feel committed to having to work on days that my disability gets the better of me. My life with Mike has progressed and we are still together but living differently as he found his own place and I live with him most of the time, but go home in the daytime to work and get picked up when Mike finishes in the evening. I think life will always be tricky, juggling my time and energy toward those I love and getting my priorities right.

The last few months have presented a number of difficult trials for me and could even be told as a further sequel to what I have been through. But for now I will keep strong and endeavour to keep on loving those that need me.